COVID-19: Inside the Global Epicenter

Personal Accounts from NYC Frontline Healthcare Providers

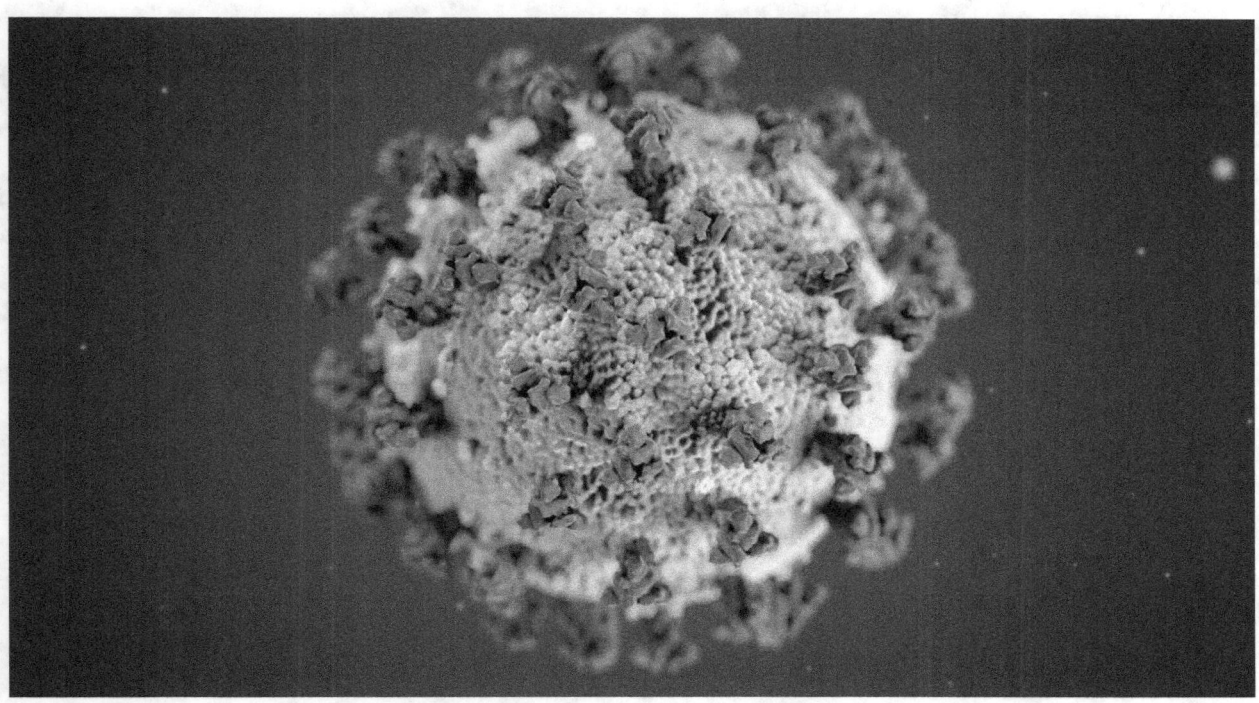

Written by Dr. Krutika Parasar Raulkar, MD
  Physical Medicine & Rehabilitation Resident

Photography by Adelene Egan, BSN, RN, CEN
  Emergency Department Nurse

TABLE OF CONTENTS

Author's Note

Photographer's Note

Timeline

Note on Layout

Chapter 1: Pandemic

- *March 16th Letter from Dr. Michael Prodromou, MD, Pulmonary Critical Care/ICU Attending Redeployed to Mt. Sinai Queens, NYC*

- *A Construct for Uncertainty—Dr. Kaile Eison, DO, Physical Medicine & Rehabilitation Resident Physician, NYC*

Chapter 2: Guilt

- *"We're all in this together"—Dr. Theodora Vamvouris, MD, Hospitalist at Yale New Haven Hospital*

- *My Husband's Death—Priya Jose, Registered Nurse, NY*

Chapter 3: Coronaviruses

- *Underreported Disability—Lorenzo Casertano, Physical Therapist, NYC*

- *Stream of Consciousness Journaling During Redeployment to the Emergency Department—Dr. Katie Rief, MD, Physical Medicine & Rehabilitation Resident Physician, NYC*

Chapter 4: Pathology of COVID-19

- *Caring for Adults with Severe Mental Illness—Catherine Migel, Licensed Clinical Social Worker and Manager of Adult Group Homes, NJ*

Chapter 5: Initial Transmission of COVID-19

- *Redeployed to the Surgical ICU—Dr. Vera Tsetlina, MD, Physical Medicine & Rehabilitation Resident Physician, NYC*
- *International Perspective: Bangalore, India—Anu and Sanjay Ganapathy, CEO of SPAN Healthcare*

Chapter 6: Comparison to Previous Pandemics

- *Reflections from the ED Crisis Unit—Dr. Jyothirmayi, PA-C, Emergency Department, Crisis Unit, Department of Psychiatry, University Hospital, Newark, NJ*
- *International Perspective: Cape Town, South Africa—Dr. Yatish Garach, MD, Gastroenterologist*

Chapter 7: Risk Factors

- *Mixed Emotions—Dr. Eugene Palatulan, MD, Physical Medicine & Rehabilitation Resident Physician Redeployed to the ED, NYC*
- *International Perspective: Singapore—Kalpa Mahender*

Chapter 8: Testing for COVID-19

- *Reflections from a Speech Language Pathologist (SLP)—Talia Schwartz, MS-CCC-SLP, NYC*
- *International Perspective: Portugal—Nandini Singla, Indian Ambassador to Portugal*

Chapter 9: Prevention of COVID-19

- *Redeployed to Queens—Dr. Michael Prodromou, MD, Pulmonary Critical Care/ICU Attending at Mt. Sinai, NYC*
- *Working on the Frontlines—Camille Culbegnan, RN, Pediatric Emergency Department, NYC*

Chapter 10: Medical Complications of COVID-19

- *Pregnancy and COVID-19—Dr. Laura Riley, MD, Chair of the Department of Obstetrics and Gynecology, NYC*
- *Treating Renal Failure from COVID-19—Dr. Revekka Babayev, MD, Nephrologist, CT*

Chapter 11: Treatments for COVID-19
- *Pediatric Emergency Medicine—Dr. Anju Wagh, MD, Pediatric Emergency Medicine Physician, NYC*
- *Getting COVID-19—Emily Jackson, Nursing Director in the Division of Medicine and Neurosciences, NYC*

Chapter 12: COVID-19 and Children
- *Giving Birth During the Pandemic—Helen Chen, mother of beautiful baby boy Harrison*
- *Homeschooling while Working from Home—Aparna Jade, Business Analyst, GA*

Chapter 13: COVID-19 in New York
- *March 24th Letter from Dr. Michael Prodromou, MD, Pulmonary Critical Care/ICU Attending Redeployed to Mt. Sinai Queens, NYC*

Chapter 14: COVID-19 in Nursing Homes
- *Caring for COVID Patients in Multiple Settings—Dr. Samuel Rosenberg, DO, Physical Medicine & Rehabilitation Attending Physician, NYC*

Chapter 15: Hospital Response to the Novel Coronavirus
- *April 7th Letter from Dr. Michael Prodromou, MD, Pulmonary Critical Care/ICU Attending Redeployed to Mt. Sinai Queens, NYC*

- *"Six degrees apart, six degrees together"—Ansel Oommen, Clinical Lab Technologist who works the night shift, NYC*

Chapter 16: COVID-19 in America

- *Redeployed to the Emergency Department—Dr. Katie Rief, MD, Physical Medicine & Rehabilitation Resident Physician, NYC*
- *International Perspective: Israel—Ronen Benhaim, VP sales of start-up company*

Chapter 17: Reopening America

- *Caring for Geriatric Patients—Dr. Gina Kang, MD, Geriatrician at Yale New Haven Hospital, CT*
- *International Perspective: Finland—Pekka Pajamo, Chief Financial Officer of Varma, a large pension insurance company*

Chapter 18: Economic Impact

- *Creating the COVID Recovery Unit—Dr. Kaile Eison, DO, Physical Medicine & Rehabilitation Resident Physician, NYC*
- *Testing and Immunity—Dr. Madhuri Tarumandas, MD, Infectious Diseases Specialist, NYC*

Chapter 19: Worldwide Impact

- *"Let's Make Sure They're Comfortable"—Dr. Osama Kandalaft, MD, Internal Medicine Hospitalist at Yale New Haven Hospital, CT*
- *COVID's Impact on Other Organ Systems—Traumatic Brain Injury Nurse Practitioner, NY*

Chapter 20: Neglect of Other Illnesses

- *New Nurse in the ICU—Julien Deshler, RN, ICU Nurse, NYC*

- *On the Proning Team—Lance DeGuzman, Occupational Therapist, NYC*

Chapter 21: Resurgence

- *Reflections from the COVID Service—Dr. Ritu Nahar, MD, Internal Medicine Resident at Jefferson University Medical Center, PA*
- *May 24th Letter from Dr. Michael Prodromou, MD, Pulmonary Critical Care/ICU Attending Redeployed to Mt. Sinai Queens, NYC*

Book Group Discussion Questions

Recommended Reading

Acknowledgements

About the Author

About the Photographer

Bibliography

In loving memory of Jose Thomas

Beloved husband, father, brother
Mental health aide who spent hours caring for COVID-19 patients
Died from COVID-19 on June 3rd, 2020

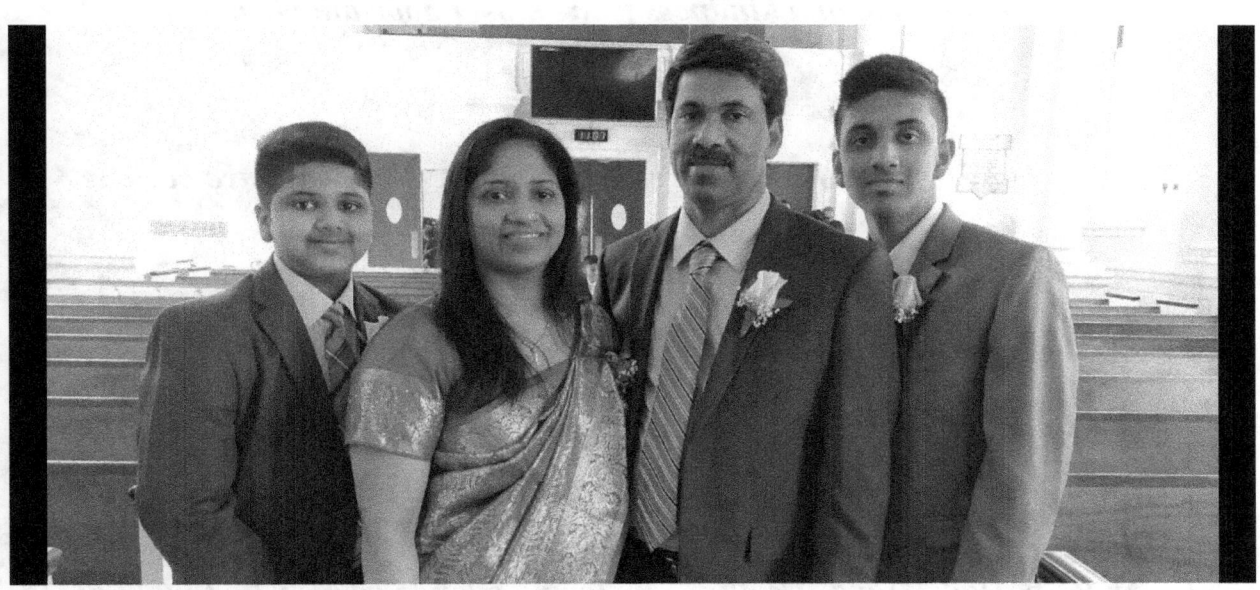

From his son: "Papa, I will really miss your beautiful smile. I will miss you taking care of us. You loved us like no other. You showed us how to love each other and how to be helpful. You never bragged about anything. Papa, you were the most amazing husband to my mom, the best father for me and Jeff, the best brother for my uncle and aunts, and most importantly, you were a man of God. When we lived in England, you would drive me to school every day and you were always there waiting for me by the end of the day. When I had no friends, you were always there for me. You were my best friend. Whenever I struggled with schoolwork, you got me through it. You went through some terrible difficulties, but your passion to support our family was always there. When we first came to America in 2011, it was a new beginning for all of us. You're the most hardworking man ever—you worked day in and day out. There would be days when you couldn't come home. You loved us so much that when you went to work you would call us every few hours to check up on us and see if we needed anything. You were the healthiest human ever. You ate healthy foods all the time, and made sure we did too. We know you are in a better place watching over us. You took care of mom like she was your own daughter. I learned a lot of things from you. You taught me and Jeff how to speak Malayalam. You raised me up with God in the center of my life. The most recent thing I learned from you was driving. I wish you had more time on Earth so you could teach me more things, but God needed you and you are now in Heaven. I promise I will fulfill your dreams and continue your legacy. I will take the best care of Amma and Jeff. Papa, I love you so much."

Dedicated to my mom, my life-long advocate and inspiration as a successful and loving working mother

To my dad, who realized medicine was the right fit for me before I did and taught me that kindness is the most important virtue

To my baby brother Josh, I am so proud of the man you have become

To Ai and Baba for your love and devotion— I could never ask for better in-laws, and we could not have got through residency without your help

To my Patti, Dadi, Dada, Thatha—my loving grandparents who taught me to read and ride a bike, raised me, and helped me raise my own kids. Patti, I will always remember that you were the first to take the time to read this book

To my husband, my greatest support and the one who most believed in this book, every day I thank my lucky stars to have you as my life partner

To my children Riaan and Risa, you are my life purpose, and I love you from the bottom of my heart

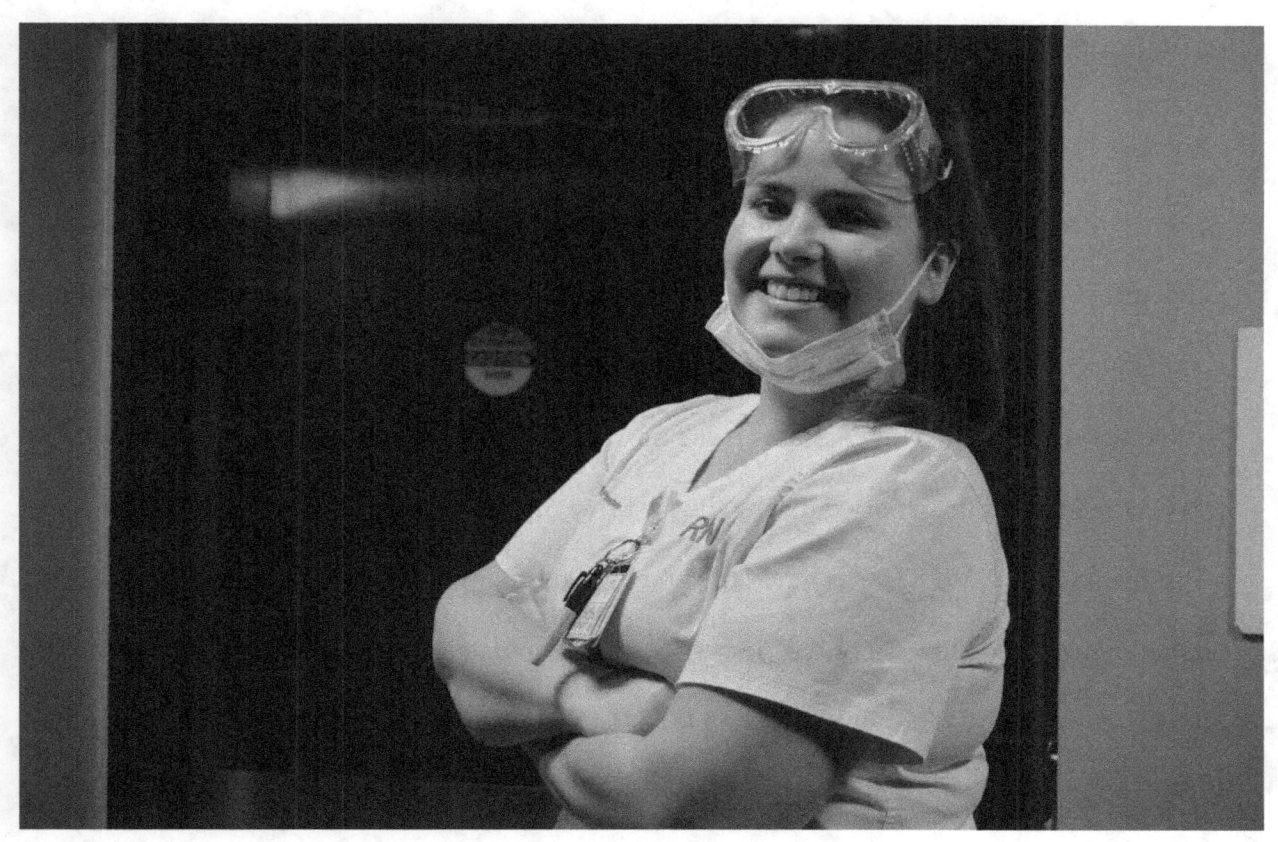

"I ask people, if they could have any superpower, what would it be. I've always said I wish I could fly, but what I didn't realize was that I've had the power to save lives all along. My community has been so amazing during this time and helped me see the beauty in my job through all the ugly. I'm actually fighting off the bad guy…COVID-19!

-Casey Fox, Registered Nurse, Emergency Department

AUTHOR'S NOTE

On March 11th 2020, the World Health Organization (WHO) declared COVID-19 a pandemic[1]. As of early August, the novel coronavirus has since infected more than 19 million and claimed the lives of over 700,000 people in more than 200 countries and territories around the world[2]. The United States is the most severely impacted nation, with over 160,000 COVID-related deaths reported during the first five months of the pandemic[2,127]. In addition to its death toll, COVID-19 has devastated the world economy, resulting in record levels of unemployment and closures of businesses. Heavily populated New York City (NYC) has been hit hardest by COVID-19, with nearly 19,000 confirmed and 5,000 probable deaths attributed to the virus[90,136]. In our final months of residency in NYC, my colleagues and I experienced the fight against the pandemic first-hand. As a rotating resident, I have had the unique opportunity and privilege to care for patients at three different hospitals during the pandemic—a private hospital that was one of the hardest hit by COVID-19, with over 750 patients ventilated in the hospital system; a free-standing rehabilitation center that cared for over 100 deconditioned and/or encephalopathic COVID patients; and a Veterans Administration (VA) hospital, part of the largest healthcare system in the country. I have seen brave essential workers put their lives on the line to care for their patients, told tearful patients and their loved ones that they are COVID-19 positive, and been shocked at the economic repercussions of the disease. This account aims to share the experiences of my colleagues and capture the devastating impact of the coronavirus at the epicenter and peak of the pandemic.

Empowered with knowledge and emboldened by camaraderie, even amidst social isolation, we will come through this. TOGETHER. In health and happiness, Dr. Krutika Parasar Raulkar

PHOTOGRAPHER's NOTE

My worlds as a nurse and photographer collided this spring when I developed my first public photo series called 'Faces of the Frontlines,' highlighting hospital personnel during the COVID-19 pandemic. This project was born out of a desire to uplift my co-workers though photography and storytelling during a trying and unprecedented moment in history. Tapping into my co-workers' personal experiences has both given me intimate access into the heart of this pandemic and strengthened my bond with and admiration for my team. Despite uncertainty about the virus and fear surrounding personal health, my co-workers show up day after day, completely prepared to give everything they can for their patients. I admire their bravery. This project has helped me process my own experience too. Being a nurse during COVID has been humbling, heartbreaking, and beautiful in some surprising ways. It helped me realize that the most important thing is just people. To be with them, to savor them, and to love them, especially when life feels super big and scary. I realized that isolation has a way of telling us that of all things, we need each other the most. The last few months have demanded our best. It has demanded that we are more resourceful, prepared, flexible, and gritty. It has asked us to stand in for our patients' families, who can't be with them. It has tested us emotionally and intellectually. I stand in awe of my colleagues who have put others ahead of themselves, making the ultimate sacrifice by risking their lives and the lives of their loved ones, to show up for other human beings when it matters most.

- Adelene Egan, RN

TIMELINE[3,4,7]:

<u>2019</u>:

November: COVID-19 thought to be transmitted from animals to humans sometime this month.

December 1st: Index case first developed symptoms of COVID-19 in Wuhan, China.

December 27th: Bronchiolar lavage of a patient from Wuhan returns positive for a new type of coronavirus.

December 30th: The Wuhan Municipal Health Commission made a public announcement to the city of a pneumonia outbreak and the first international report was released.

December 31st: The U.S. CDC learns of 27 cases of pneumonia in Wuhan from a novel coronavirus.

<u>2020</u>:

January 4th: WHO publicizes discovery of a cluster of pneumonia cases in Wuhan.

January 20th: WHO reports first confirmed cases of COVID-19 outside of China in Thailand, Japan, and South Korea.

January 23rd: First laboratory confirmed case in the United States in a 60-year-old female woman in Illinois, who returned from a trip to Wuhan, China in mid-January.

January 30th: WHO reports more than 7,000 cases in 18 countries and classifies the outbreak as a global health emergency.

January 31st: Case of COVID-19 in a man in his 30s in Washington State.

January 23rd: China quarantines people of Wuhan.

February 2nd: Temporary ban placed on travel from China by several countries, including the U.S., New Zealand, South Korea, the Philippines, Vietnam, Indonesia, Hong Kong, Japan and Maldives. Most allowed their own citizens to return to their countries.

February 7th: Li Wenliang, a 34-year-old ophthalmologist at Wuhan Central Hospital, dies from complications of COVID-19. He was one of 8 doctors who tried to share information about COVID-19 when it was discovered, but was reprimanded by Wuhan police for his efforts.

February 16th: Hubei institutes a "hard quarantine" of its people allowing only one person to leave each household for a limited time every three days to obtain provisions.

March 11th: WHO declares COVID-19 a pandemic.

March 27th: President Trump signed the Coronavirus Aid, Relief, and Economic Security (CARES) Act, which provided a $2.2 trillion aid package that included direct stimulus payments.

April 23rd: NYC antibody testing reveals that 21.2 % of residents tested were positive for COVID-19.

April 24th: Georgia begins to reopen gyms and fitness centers and nail, massage, hair, and tattoo parlors.

May 2nd: Nearly 40,000 cases and 1,700 deaths due to COVID-19 in Africa, with 53 African countries affected.

May 11th: China reports first new cluster of cases since Wuhan's lockdown was removed[28].

May 12th: The United States continues to have the highest caseload of COVID-19, followed by Russia[28].

May 15th: New York State starts reopening up-state counties.

May 18th: More than 100 countries have petitioned the World Health Assembly to investigate the WHO's management of the coronavirus pandemic[28].

May 20th: China reports new cluster of cases with longer recovery time, suggesting that the virus could be mutating[72].

June 1st: Eli Lilly studies using monoclonal antibodies as a treatment for COVID-19. Chief scientist notes that treatment could be available as early as September[126].

June 8th: New York City starts to reopen.

June 10th: U.S. case load reaches 2 million[130].

June 16th: The U.S. Department of Health and Safety announced that a COVID-19 vaccine would be free for patients at highest risk for COVID-19 who could not otherwise afford it[130].

June 18th: The WHO stops hydroxychloroquine trial due to lack of beneficiary evidence[130].

July 11th: Disney World reopens two of its theme parks despite increasing cases in Florida. Strict crowd control, mask requirements, and temperature and bag checks are in place[131].

Disclaimer:

The content in this book is meant for informational purposes only and does not constitute medical advice.

Note on Layout:

This book aims to shed light on COVID-19 through multiple formats.

First, each chapter provides historical and and/or medical information regarding the pandemic, infused with my personal experiences. This aims to educate and inform with broad content in a readable format. Prior to each chapter is a quote, either from John M. Barry's *The Great Influenza,* or a figure involved in the response against the coronavirus.

Second, each chapter includes quotes and/or photos of frontline workers captured by Adelene Egan, BSN, RN, CEN. Her brilliant photography captures the optimism and camaraderie that existed during the pandemic—universal sentiment felt by all providers with whom I spoke.

Third, each chapter features the personal accounts of frontline workers. I cannot express how much I have enjoyed speaking with each and every one of these healthcare heroes—and how thankful I am that they are willing to share their stories with the world. They are truly the life and blood of this book, and the reason that thousands of COVID-19 related deaths have been prevented.

CHAPTER 1: PANDEMIC

"Pandemic is not a word to be used lightly or carelessly. It is a word that, if misused, can cause unreasonable fear, or unjustified acceptance that the fight is over, leading to unnecessary suffering and death."

- Dr. Tedros Adhanom, WHO director general[65]

On March 3rd, 2020, we gathered in our conference room for a journal club regularly scheduled with Dr. Joel Stein, the Chair of the Department of Rehabilitation and Regenerative Medicine. I was mentally rehearsing my presentation of an article on the benefits of high intensity stepping for inpatient stroke survivors. As kind and approachable as Dr. Stein is, it is nevertheless daunting to present in front of our erudite department chair. I was about to launch into my presentation, when Dr. Stein said he had an important announcement to make. Our hospital had its first case of COVID-19. Dr. Stein speaks with calm and compassion as he delivers this pronouncement. He expects a pandemic. He says this could reach the proportions of the 1918 Spanish influenza.

I am shocked by this last statement. Over the past months I have seen articles on the coronavirus peppering the New York Times and my FlipIt app, but I often scroll through looking for articles on exercise, nutrition, parenting—my go-to topics. Now that COVID-19 is in our city, in our hospital, it becomes real.

Dr. Stein goes on to say that institution-related travel has been banned, so the American Academy of Physical Medicine and Rehabilitation conference scheduled this weekend in Florida has been cancelled. Faces around the room look disappointed. Our residents have been waiting all year to attend this conference. For some it is their opportunity to present research and their annual vacation. Little did we know that something so important to us at the time would pale in comparison to the devastating impact of COVID-19 in the months to come.

After journal club, my co-residents and I regrouped in the resident room to tend to admission and discharge paperwork, consult notes—the mounting pile of documentation that is a bulk of medical practice. The resident room buzzed with speculation and questions regarding the coronavirus and what it would mean for us— what it would mean for New York and the rest of the world. My co-resident with asthma questioned whether he should wear a mask at all times. He later would be reprimanded for doing so, told that he was using precious personal protective equipment (PPE) inappropriately. His father eventually developed a severe case of COVID-19 requiring prolonged intubation. Thankfully, he recovered and is now walking with decreasing oxygen requirements. At the forefront of my thoughts is my 55-year-old asthmatic father who commutes daily to Manhattan, where New York's first COVID-19 patient also worked.

During the early days of the pandemic I was rotating at as a consult physiatry resident. To rapidly increase its force of healthcare workers, New York granted emergency licenses to practice medicine in the state. Fourth year medical students were allowed to graduate a few months early so they could enter residency and fight the virus. Retired physicians were requested to return to work to assist in the battle. This immediate and composed response to the virus was essential to care for the onslaught of thousands of COVID-19 patients, the majority of whom were eventually discharged home with their families. The country rallied together to fight the virus, and as horrifying as the toll has been, the number of cases has not yet approached experts' estimates of a death rate approaching 200,000 people in the United States.

What is the coronavirus? How did it originate? How did the country and world handle its discovery and rapid spread? Who is getting affected? What treatments are available? I decided to write this book after an evening conversation with my 63-year-old neighbor, Susan. We stood more than six feet apart in the hallway of our apartment and her COVID-related questions spilled out. She was concerned about the virus's impact on her and even more so on her adult children, one of whom takes immunosuppressive medications after a kidney transplant. Susan was the donor. Over the next hour, I answered her questions and she was so thankful for our conversation. I realized that many people could benefit from information concerning the virus in a readable, unpartisan format. And so, this book began.

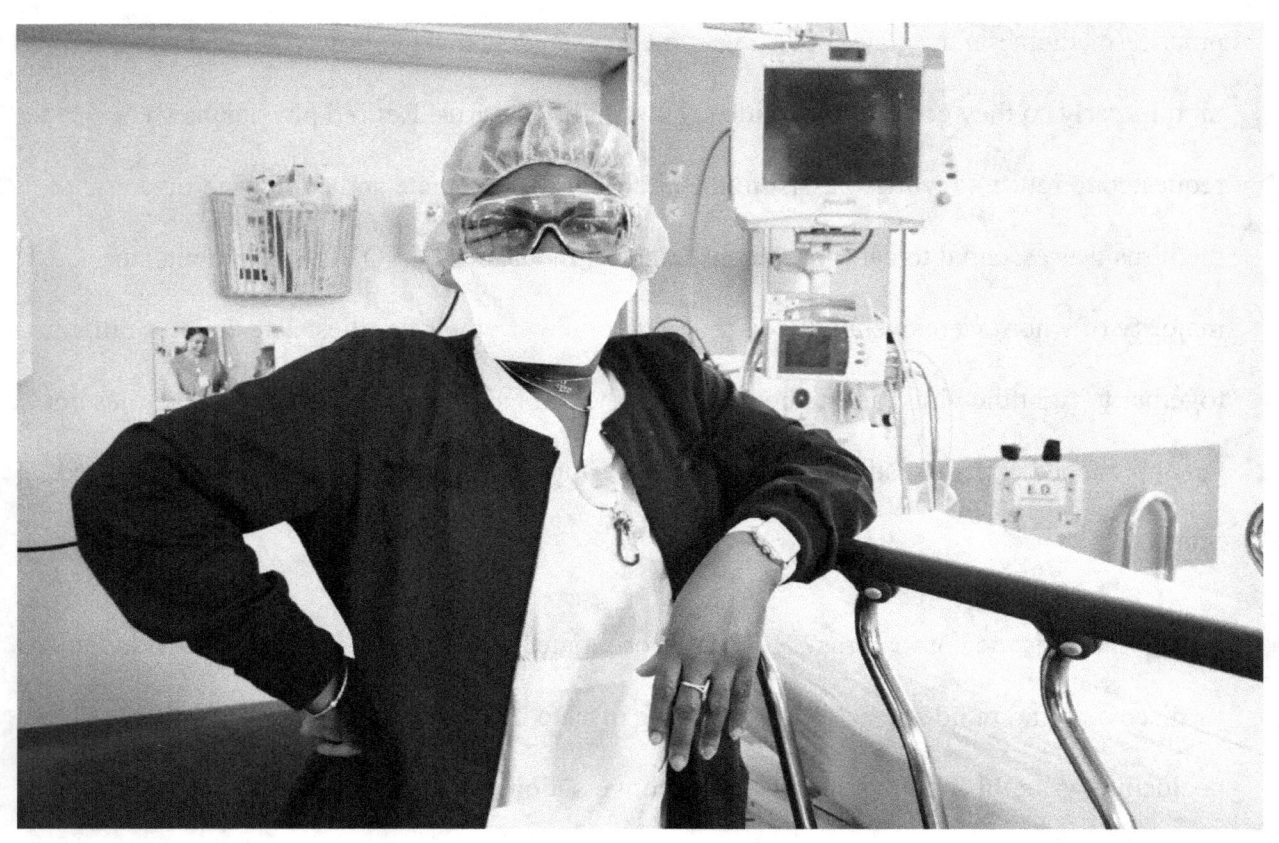

"I am on the battlefield."

-Rose Davis, Registered Nurse, Emergency Department, NYC

A Construct for Uncertainty

-Dr. Kaile Eison, DO, Physical Medicine & Rehabilitation Resident Physician, NYC

Texts from my husband:

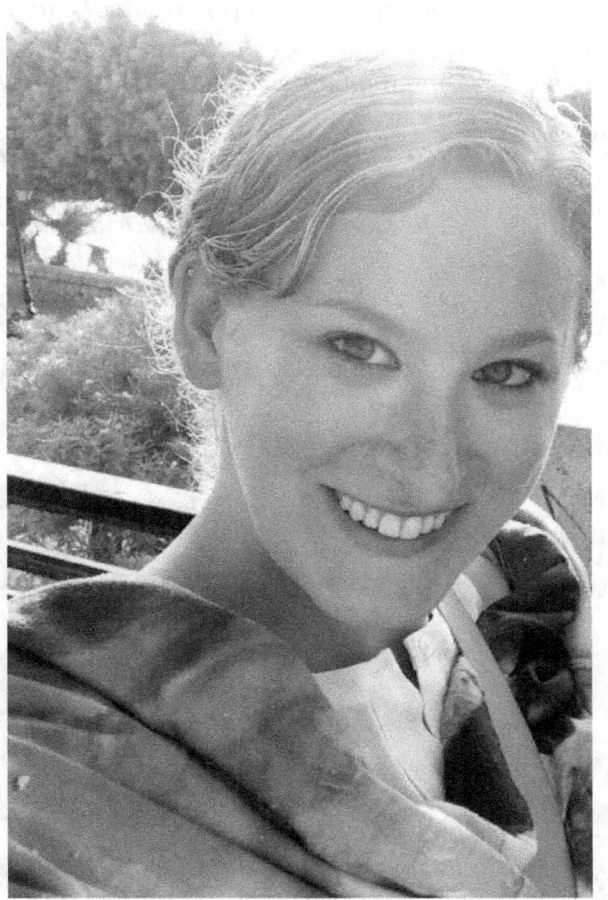

Thursday 1:18pm: Calling us for resp distress. Asking if we should be concerned for covid. Not really sure. Doesn't have any risk factors but idk.

5:08pm: Wondering if I should take extra precautions if we tube.

Friday 7:21am: I'm being emergently credentialed as an attending in the ED!

Saturday 12:34pm: They just cancelled my oral boards.

Sunday 6:18am: Another covid rule out.

Monday 3:08pm: Cleared out the surgical patients for covid overflow.

Tuesday 6:29am: Almost out of N95s. Gonna have to reuse them.

Wednesday 11:40am: Every icu is turning into a covid icu.

Thursday 6:48am: 2 covid positive codes overnight. No real way to protect ourselves. It's really bad.

Today 5:49pm: Almost out of vents…

I didn't start out thinking I was going to be a physician. I was going to be an actor. I committed myself to a life of emotional expression, artistic fulfillment, and likely poverty, and pursued an undergraduate conservatory degree in theater, which I quickly found is one of the most nebulous forms of education one can obtain. Rolling around on the floor, drawing classmates nude, and learning to imagine hot coffee in an empty cup were all part of a curriculum crafted to create the ideal artist. As an actor, there is relatively little structure or guidance, and there are almost never definitive answers. Much of the time, the emotion one feels and that which can be conveyed to an audience is more valuable an answer than simple mathematics or a binary solution to a problem. I was taught to strip down to my most vulnerable in order to learn and experience my most basic, rawest truth. I asked myself difficult questions, soul-searching daily in order to find not an answer, but a human representation of the struggle and search that is common and relatable to all people. There are no "yes or no" questions in acting, and so the actor lives forever in uncertainty. And when I decided that I would always love acting, but that I no longer wanted to pursue it as a career, a portion of my decision was because I wanted to know not only from where my next paycheck would come, but also because I was tired of the extreme subjectivity of everything within the field. I didn't want that uncertainty.

I chose to become a physician because I asked too many "whys". I wanted to know why things were the way they were, why a character -- a person -- behaved or moved in the way that he or she did. I wanted to understand people and, rather than put that on stage, use *it to help them. And get answers, I did. In medical school, I learned to retrain my brain to understand that pathologies have pathways and medications have mechanisms and people die because something somewhere shuts down and we can track it to that very chemical moment. Questions had answers and science was made up of facts. But the longer I've been a physician, the more I've realized that, despite our answers, we make a practice of living with uncertainty. Deciding when to watch and when to take action. Picking which treatment plan is going to help and which is going to harm. Predicting whether or not a patient's paretic limb function will return or whether they will walk again. Choosing when to tell a patient's family to come in because their loved one probably isn't going to make it through the night. Now, more than ever, we live in times of uncertainty. I'm married to an emergency medicine-critical care doctor. He is on the front lines, for lack of a better term, of the COVID-19 pandemic. He is exposed on a daily basis. He will likely start to show symptoms at some point. Every morning, I tell him to be safe, as if somehow saying it will make a difference. And here I am, a physiatrist, waiting, as physiatrists do, for the downstream effects. For patients to be transferred to clear beds. For them to survive long enough to make it to the floor. For my husband to get sick. For me to be exposed. For the world to keep shutting down. For things to get better. As I wait, I find myself thinking back to my training as an actor. It's my construct for uncertainty. It is forcing me to be alright with not having the answers. And I suppose, in some ways, the not knowing is the art of medicine. It is the vulnerability that makes us, as physicians, human.*

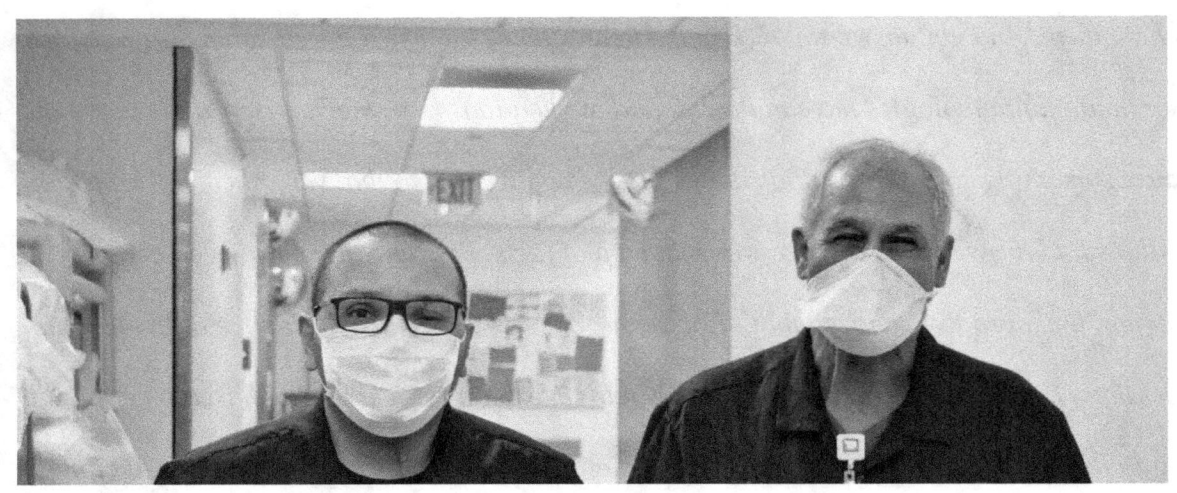

"How are you home girl? If you're good, I'm good home girl."

-Roberto Toro & Carlos Garcia, Environmental Services, NYC

Letter from Michael Prodromou, Pulmonary Critical Care/ICU Attending Redeployed to Mt. Sinai Queens, NYC

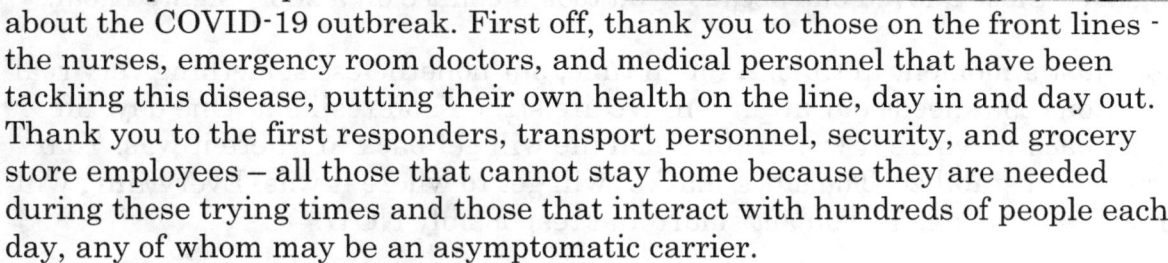

March 16th:

To my dear friends and family,
I feel compelled to put in a few words about the COVID-19 outbreak. First off, thank you to those on the front lines - the nurses, emergency room doctors, and medical personnel that have been tackling this disease, putting their own health on the line, day in and day out. Thank you to the first responders, transport personnel, security, and grocery store employees – all those that cannot stay home because they are needed during these trying times and those that interact with hundreds of people each day, any of whom may be an asymptomatic carrier.

Never in my wildest dreams would I imagine dealing with something that seems to be straight out of a sci-fi horror movie. Restaurants brimming with life are now desolate and abandoned. At the grocery store, I see empty frozen food sections, and a sea of purple gloves and surgical masks. It's a different world.

In every aspect of life, extremes are never the answer. Amongst the life threatening and dangerous potential of COVID-19, we are worsening the situation by turning on ourselves – finger pointing about not being prepared, people that refuse to understand the gravity of the situation, businesses actually weighing corporate greed against people's health and wellbeing, panic, hysteria, people looking out for themselves and nobody else.

Don't blame one political figure for being grossly underprepared – right or not, politics aside, it's not about what happened, it's about what to do NOW. Don't come to me and remind me that at one point the medical community said, "Oh the flu is more dangerous, worry about that more," or ask me "How can you not have a cure or vaccine for this?" I'm sorry that we don't actually have the answer immediately upon the presentation of a new bug like COVID-19. Nature changes. Science changes. Guidelines change. We get it, it's frustrating to be the patient hearing mixed signals.

This is not the time to be ignorant. A simple measure such as social distancing can help immensely. I know we have to change the way we live for a little bit. It sucks, but it must be done. Businesses will lose money. People will lose money. Life will be a little bit more difficult. I hope we agree that people's lives, of those you love or don't even know, are most important right now. So many organizations and businesses have suspended or restricted their operations for the wellbeing of their employees – I appreciate their sacrifice – much respect. If you are a business that is still, despite all the recommendations of our medical experts, insisting on carrying out nonessential duties and not looking out for the health and safety of your employees, SHAME on you.

Stay home. It's inconvenient and it sucks. However, it can save lives. Not just yours, but all your loved ones that may be a little bit more vulnerable. Don't give into the panic and hysteria, and don't give this virus the fuel it needs to keep it going. Don't lose a loved one because you took a chance on a short-sighted goal.

This is just a moment in time. A tough time, but nonetheless something very real and serious that needs our attention. We are strong and resilient. One day, life will get back to where it was. Your social life will get back to where it was. Your finances will stabilize. The stock market will get to where it was. Everything will correct itself, so long as you act smart and responsibly NOW.

I let the panic and hysteria get to me. This past weekend I ran into Whole Foods, without a cart or basket because I was so concerned about getting coronavirus from the handles. I basically grabbed everything my two arms could hold and headed for the register. After 20 minutes waiting online, I started losing my grip. Items began to drop. People had to help me pick things up. The lady behind me asked me if I wanted to share her shopping cart. At any point in time, this would have been seen as a small gesture, but given the circumstances, I was struck by her selflessness. Panic can make us do stupid things. It can isolate us, and divided we lose.

We need to work together against COVID-19 – we need to make sacrifices such as social distancing, we need to watch out for our most vulnerable, and not be selfish. Together we will overcome. Together we will make life return to normal. Give it time, give it patience, and be smart about your actions.

Let's stand together against COVID-19 (each in the safety of our own homes…)

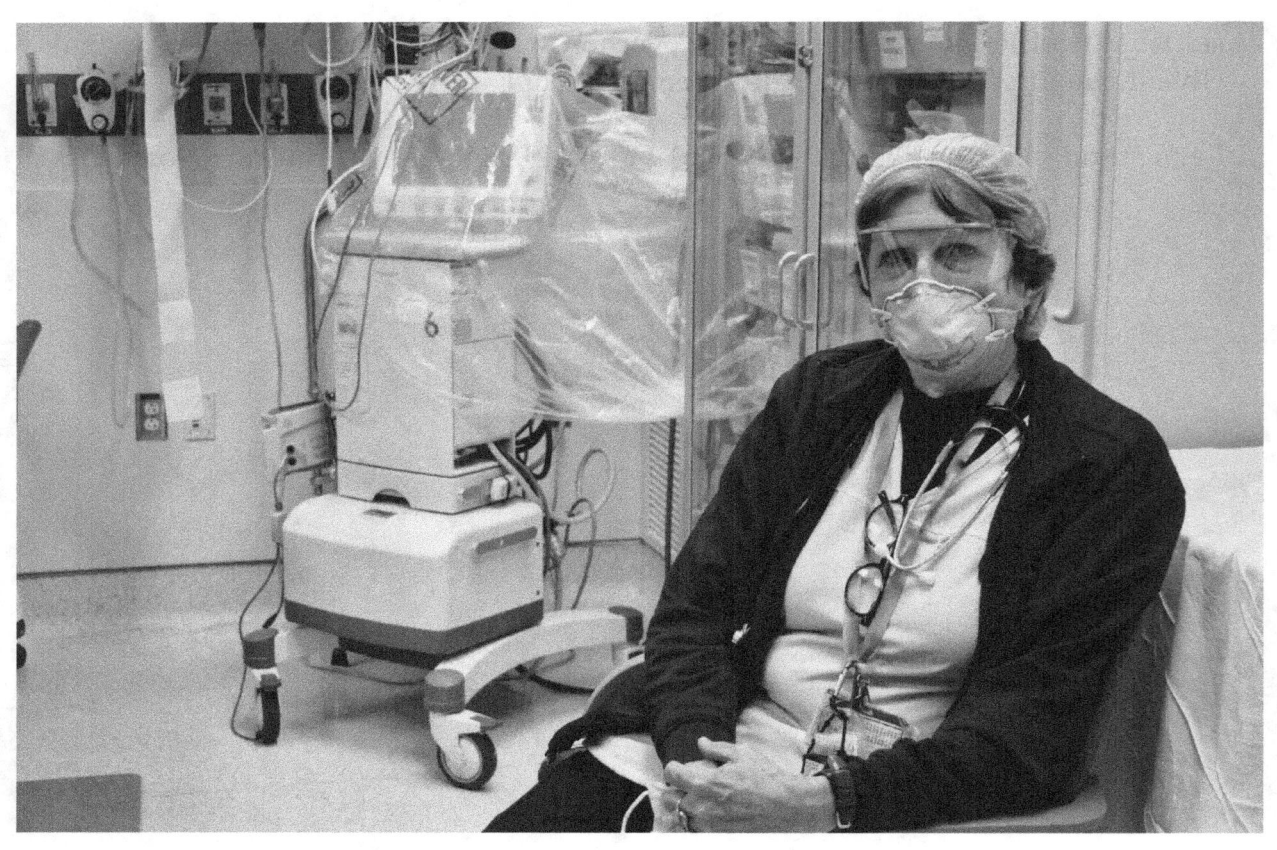

"To achieve success, you need a recipe of ingredients. Everything you put in will only lead to a great outcome. During this difficult time, we have learned a lot about ourselves and tested our coping mechanisms. I am so proud to work with all of you and refer to you as family. Keep smiling behind your masks, the glimmer in your eyes shows your kindness."

-Marie Owens, Registered Nurse, Emergency Department, NYC

CHAPTER 2: GUILT

"Finding useful material on the epidemic proved remarkably difficult. It was easy enough to find stories of death, but my own interests have always focused on people who try to exercise some kind of control over events. Anyone doing so was far too busy, far to overwhelmed, to pay any attention to keeping records."

-John M. Barry in *The Great Influenza*

When the pandemic started, I vehemently wanted to volunteer to be on the front lines with colleagues. Rehabilitation Medicine typically serves in both the outpatient and inpatient arenas. While our inpatient facilities experienced high demand during the pandemic, our outpatient facilities were relegated to telemedicine visits in the first two months. Outpatient residents were homebound, bored, and restless as the city hunkered down and they were unable to help like our counterparts in the EDs and ICUs. This rapidly changed as the need for healthcare workers grew, and all outpatient residents were soon redeployed to the EDs, ICUs, COVID recovery units, and additional inpatient rehabilitation units—busier than they ever imagined.

Throughout the pandemic I was always deployed—first on the rehabilitation medicine consult service, then in a Traumatic Brain Injury Unit at a free-standing rehabilitation hospital, and finally in a VA Spinal Cord Injury unit. I was able to care for COVID positive veterans and traumatic brain injury patients suffering from long term critical illness myopathy, neuropathy and encephalopathy due to the disease. However, most of my patient care during this time was devoted to COVID negative patients, whom we tried to isolate from COVID positive patients to avoid disease spread. I felt guilty that I was not in the trenches with my co-residents, who were overwhelmed with COVID patients. At the same time, I live in a one-bedroom apartment with my husband, elderly in-laws, and two children. While I had little fear for my husband and my children, my in-laws are at risk of severe infection given their age. Was it right for me to volunteer for redeployment and put my family at risk? Furthermore, non-COVID patients still desperately needed care and as an increasing amount of resources and healthcare providers were being re-directed to the COVID effort, my patients needed me more than ever. The fact that they were alone in the hospital without visitors made them especially vulnerable, isolated, and at risk for mental health disorders.

    Looking back, I am so thankful for my experiences in all three hospitals where I worked during the pandemic. Caring for both COVID and non-COVID patients during this time has been a life experience I will never forget. No matter what unit we were on or which patients we cared for, we lived and breathed COVID-19—constantly researching, conversing, sharing experiences and knowledge about the disease and both its acute and chronic manifestations, and always at risk of contracting the virus and spreading it to our loved ones and neighbors. I have utmost admiration for my colleagues who braved the bulk of the storm, flattening the curve, and rescuing so many patients from this deadly disease. This book is a testament to their bravery and I am proud to be able to share their experiences with the world.

We're all in this together

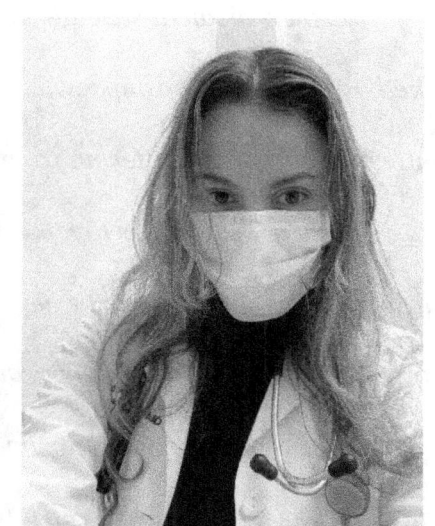

-*Theodora Vamvouris, MD, Hospitalist at Yale New Haven Hospital, CT*

What was it like to work at Yale during the peak of the pandemic? *Our peak COVID-19+ patient load was 450, and we are currently at 200. Of the 450, about 70 required ventilators and about 100 required ICU care. I have often covered and admitted hospital floor patients who would deteriorate and require transfer to the ICU for intubation. Covering COVID positive patients was always scary as their status could change rapidly, requiring quick transition to a higher level of care.*

What was the camaraderie like on your unit? *The camaraderie is the most comforting and touching part of working during this crisis. It feels as though I am working with true friends rather than co-workers and that certainly sweetens the bitterness of the pandemic. One night after covering seven rapid responses, one of my co-workers thoughtfully offered to take care of one to ease my burden, and that meant so much to me. Also, the pleasant company and laughs we share make the world of difference. We are there for each other to vent about our experiences, and share our fears and frustrations, which mostly revolve around fears of running out of PPE and being exposed. I often joked that I was in greater danger of being* *poisoned from the extensive sterilization than suffering from COVID itself, and it felt reassuring to share this with my co-worker friends.*

Further, medical specialists went beyond their scopes of practice and enthusiastically helped us. Our relationships with nurses grew stronger. We supported our co-workers whose family members were suffering from COVID by contributing to collective gifts. Colorful signs reading "We are all in this together" adorned with hearts and happiness touched me deeply. Our local community was also supportive, making us accessories with love to show their appreciation. We are all deeply grateful!

I feel so humbled and fortunate by our administrative support. We have bi-weekly virtual meetings to safely and openly discuss our experiences and challenges and to stay informed and updated on the most current trends and treatments. Specialists such as hematologists and cardiologists often join our meetings and engage in discussions on treating this new and unfamiliar disease. Our institution had a plan and this gave us confidence. Most of all, they are compassionate. Hospitalists at increased risk due to their age or comorbidities were not assigned to patients with COVID-19, and that made me so proud to be a part of the Yale community, where we look out for each other not just as doctors but as human beings.

Do you have any patient experiences that most affected you? *A physician-patient relationship is sacred and this is no different with a patient suffering from COVID. However, this illness creates an emotional barrier of fear along with a cold physical barrier of PPE. This further alienates us from our patients and makes it so much more difficult to carry out our role of comforting and getting to know the person we are treating rather than the disease he or she carries. I'd feel guilty of the lingering fear that would challenge my focus on their* *ailments. I'd try my best to hold their hands with my gloved ones and connect with them through my full-face respirator in hope of offering comfort during their times of distress. Human connection is such a large part of being a physician, and* this has become so much more challenging with COVID.

Were there any treatments that you found to be effective? *Assessing treatment efficacy is difficult outside a controlled trial. We have not noticed significant benefit from hydroxychloroquine and have now stopped using it as we found its cardiac risks outweigh any benefits. I may have seen some benefit with tocilizumab, but this can't be confirmed as it has not been compared to a control. There is a remdesivir trial at Yale, and its use shows strong promise in the literature.*

What would you like people to know about COVID-19? *COVID-19 is a new, life-impacting experience for all of us, whether we are in healthcare or not. We have all been significantly thrown off our routines and isolated from one another. My partner lives long distance, and I have been unable to see him for over three months. If he were to stay with me, I'd have the burden of possibly passing the disease to him and causing him harm and this has greatly affected me. Further, the comfort of visiting friends has been contaminated by the fear of contracting or passing a dangerous virus. One of my friends fractured her arm, and I feel so bad for her as she is suffering in isolation devoid of physical comfort. Touch is a significant part of human comfort and we are robbed of this. We have been asked to forego an essential part of being human because to be human is to be social and this disease has plagued us with social isolation. As a doctor, I hold both the privilege and burden of stepping out of social* *isolation in hope of living up to the Hippocratic Oath. This virus has emphasized that we are "all in this together" whether we are a doctor or nurse directly caring for patients, a grocery store clerk maintaining our vitality, or a teenager fighting against their social nature and staying home to ensure that their families and their neighbors stay safe.*

Never in our worst nightmares would we have expected to be practicing medicine with the fear of running out of PPE and sterilizing solution. I have bought my own surgical masks, alcohol, and respirators, as I am afraid of running out. Thanks to overpriced eBay masks, I can use more than one surgical mask per shift and trial different, safe, re-useable respirators, while easing some of the PPE burden at our hospital. I believe that we should have been more prepared for this as a nation and that people in healthcare should have the ability to buy their own equipment online directly through manufacturers' websites rather than anxiously purchasing masks on eBay. And I say this with a feeling of gratitude and advantage, as our hospital has gone above and beyond to supply us with PPE, but there is only so much they can do with the national shortage. We need to be better prepared as a nation should we face something like this again.

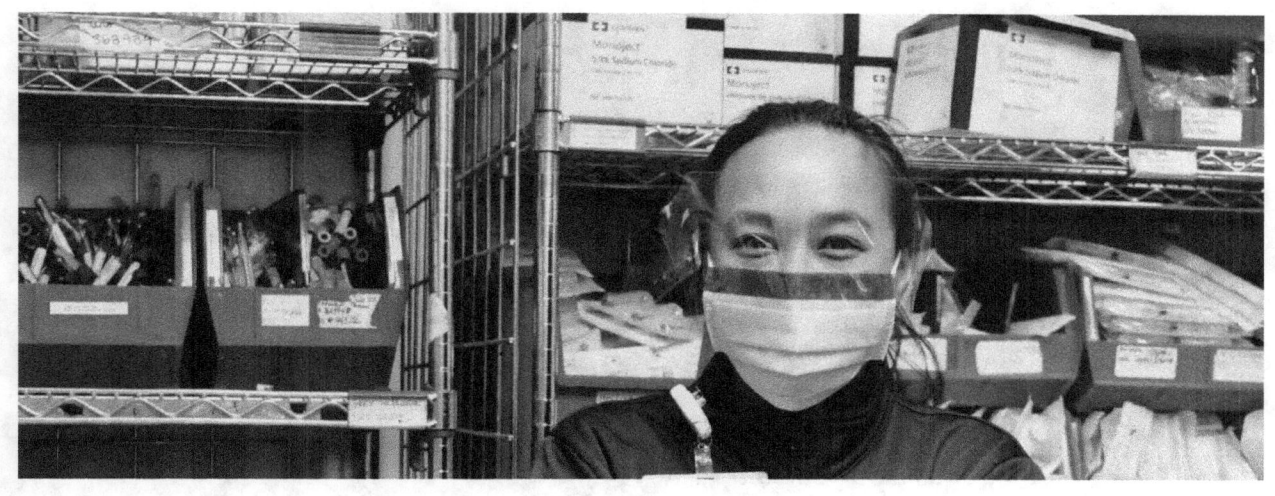

"Many describe the ED as busy, scary, emotional, hopeful, unpredictable…we relate to it as our home away from home. My ED family continues to inspire and impress me. A heartfelt THANK YOU to our everyday heroes."

-Christel Vasquez, Registered Nurse, Emergency Department & Patient Care Director, NYC

My Husband's Death

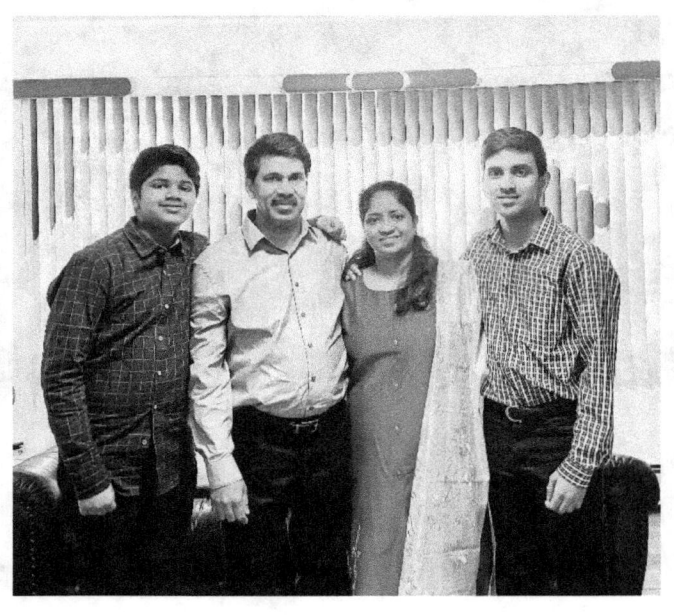

Priya Jose, Registered Nurse, NY

My husband was a 53-year-old man who worked full-time as a mental health aide. He was a hardworking man, with shifts from 3:30pm to 12am, and was very dedicated to his patients. He was on the frontline caring for COVID-19 patients. I work as a nurse at the same hospital during the day shift. Early in the pandemic, we were not provided enough PPE. On April 3rd, I experienced symptoms of Covid-19 and my husband was tested negative. This was possibly a false reading. He went to work as per protocol.

That week, he was working with a severely ill COVID positive patient with whom he was with for 16 hours. Proper PPE was still unavailable at our hospital. The next day he went shopping and started shivering. He experienced a high fever that night. The next morning, he was found to be positive. He had no symptoms other than fever. The doctor said to stay home from work for 14 days. He continued to have high fever for about 3-4 days. While working in the hospital, we saw that a lot of people were getting pneumonia, and so we thought it was best to go to urgent care to rule out this complication. The x-ray results showed bilateral pneumonia, and he received an oral antibiotic and returned home. His fever resolved, but after three days he developed a sensation that something was stuck in the middle of his chest.

He still had no shortness of breath or body pain and no longer had fever. He thought maybe it was phlegm and we tried to flush it out with hot drinks and steam inhalation.

I made soup for him but he did not have an appetite. I asked him if he wanted to return to the doctor, but he said, "No, I'm ok, I have no shortness of breath or dyspnea." My brother-in-law brought a pulse oximeter, and he was saturating at 92-94%. I kept checking, and his saturations remained at these levels. At that time, we were unaware that COVID patients had increased risk of blood clots. Something continued to bother him deep inside his chest and his saturation dropped to 88-90. I remember he was listening to a Christian spirituality station…I checked his saturation level and it had dropped to 84. I said we shouldn't wait here, we should go to the hospital. He said, "I feel a little weak, I want to lie down." He rested in the prone position. His sat dropped to 79. I did not call the ambulance, I quickly drove him to urgent care.

He looked like a normal person when he walked into the clinic. I told them his oxygen saturation is dropping, they called him inside and an ambulance came for him. He received 3-4 L oxygen via nasal cannula. His D-Dimer level came back elevated at 7.8. and he was started on IV antibiotics for pneumonia—doxycycline, ceftriaxone, meropenem—and started on lovenox for anticoagulation. He received 1 unit of plasma, 5 days of an anti-viral injection, and Vitamin C supplementation. On his third day in the hospital his doctor said he was doing well and I wanted to take him home. He still had a low oxygen saturation of 90, but no other issues. However, he was started on a heparin drip and had to be monitored. His chest pain resolved, and all labs were normal except for the elevated D-Dimer. It slowly trended downward—5.8, 2.8, normal. The heparin was stopped. But he was still desaturating on high flow oxygen. He was very anxious that he saw so little of his providers in the hospital, and he felt very lonely away from his family. On May 11th, the doctor called me at 4pm to tell me that he was stable. I asked, "When did you see him?" He said at 9:30 am. I said, "He just called me and told me they are planning to intubate him." His status had changed since that morning and the doctor was unaware. Later on, the doctor felt it was better to intubate him as he was becoming dyspneic and his oxygen saturation was dropping. During that entire time, my husband was talking to me on FaceTime. He was worried that he would be intubated and he would never come back. I tried to reassure him, saying "We don't want ARDS to develop, we want to let your lungs rest." He was fully alert and oriented at the time.

After intubation, he was proned, then paralyzed, because he was struggling while sedated. When transitioned from prone to supine, his breathing tube was dislodged, and from that moment his condition deteriorated. His vital signs plummeted, he became tachypneic. He went into respiratory arrest. He survived and continued on the ventilator for another two weeks. One day I called the doctor and he told me he was a stable patient and they were hoping to reduce the sedation. The next day I called and they told me he was deteriorating. I went to the hospital and he had already passed away due to cardiac arrest. The doctor never explained this to me. No one called me and I had to find out from a nurse.

The doctor had informed me he was stable and I told the doctor that if I see him, maybe he will get better. Especially during this time, my husband had no one there and he felt alone. He was very upset, anxious, and fearful when the nurse quickly informed him that he was to be intubated. I want to emphasize that it is vital for the interdisciplinary team to be kind and comforting to their patients when they are alone and sick. I am 100% sure that my *husband would still be here if I was with him. This was the first time my husband was ever admitted to the hospital. If I was there, my husband would not have been ventilated. I have regret that because of me this happened. I was able to visit him, hold his hand, and talk to him for 4 hours. Although he was not able to talk, there were tears rolling down his cheeks and I knew he could hear me. The second and last time I went, I was only allowed to stay for 30 minutes. If only I was able to hold his hands again, I believe a difference could have been made. For 1 month, my husband was away from myself and our kids. Our children couldn't see their dad and he died before they could see him again.*

When I called to ask about my husband, I was asked, "Are you a physician?" I told them no, but it is my right to ask about my husband. At least they could have told me when there was no hope. I had promised him he would come out. They told me he would survive because he is healthy. I still feel that he is on vacation. I cannot even think that he is not in this world.

I know in the hospital they don't spend much time with COVID patients. They are worried about spreading the disease and being affected by the disease themselves. As a nurse, I treated COVID patients with no PPE. One of my patients was an elderly woman—I treated her as if she was my own grandmother. I worked closely with her and that may be why I was affected by COVID, but I had to do everything I could to take care of my patients. We see the devastation in the media, but we do not actually realize what the patient and their family is going through. When it comes to your own family, you see the agony and unbearable pain.

He was a lovely husband and lovely father. My son Joel says he took care of me as if I am his daughter. He was very involved in our children's lives, such as helping them with their homework, projects, etc. Unfortunately, he passed away a week before our son's high school graduation. My son said he didn't want to go to his Commencement ceremony, since his father couldn't be there. But I told him that his father would want him to go, and he will always be watching him from Heaven. I feel I have to go from this world as soon as possible so I can be with him. My family tells me not to think that way, and I have to be strong to take care of my kids. I know my husband would want me to be happy. It hurt him to see me sad or crying.

He was a God-fearing man and had a positive way of interacting with every person. If you had the privilege of meeting him, you would never forget him, his golden smile, and bubbly personality. He has touched a lot of lives and will forever live in our hearts. He loved going to church and he never failed to tell our kids about who God is and how great he is. He always made prayer a priority every single day and as a family we always prayed on our knees while holding hands. He was always one to be positive and encouraging. Even though life was challenging at times, he always kept his faith and knew that God would come through. However, God has called him home, to the place where there is no suffering.

"I have fought the good fight, I have finished the race, I have kept the faith."

-2 Timothy 4:7-

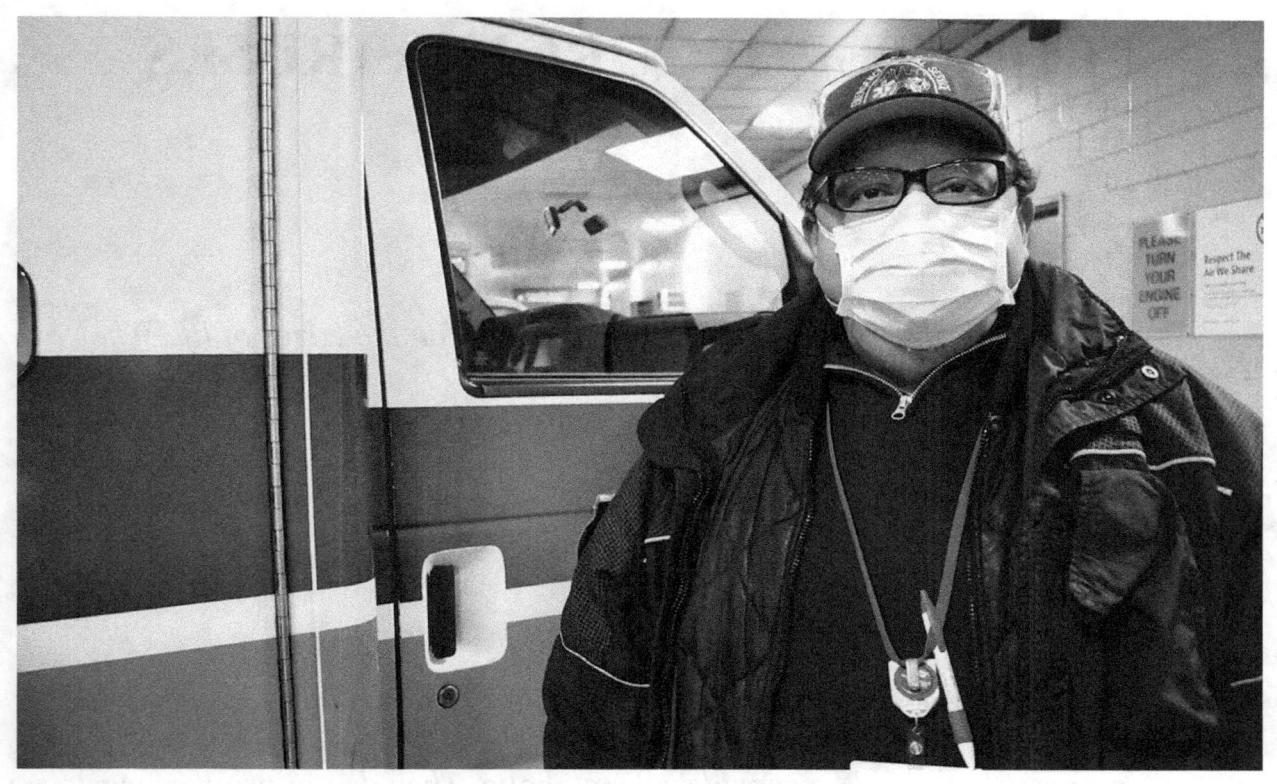

"As first responders, we leave our families with the hope not to bring a deadly virus back home at the end of our workday. We know what is needed out here and the public needs us now more than ever."

-Juan Aguirre, Paramedic, NYC

CHAPTER 3: CORONAVIRUSES

"Viruses themselves are an enigma that exist on the edges of life. They are not simply small bacteria. Bacteria consists of only one cell, but they are fully alive. Each has a metabolism, requires food, produces waste, and reproduces by division.

Viruses do not eat or burn oxygen for energy. They do not engage in any process that could be considered metabolic. They do not produce waste. They do not have sex. They make no side products, by accident or design. They do not even reproduce independently. They are less than a fully living organism but more than an inert collection of chemicals."

-John M. Barry in *The Great Influenza*

Coronaviruses (CoV) are a large family of enveloped, positive-sense, single-strand RNA viruses[13] that typically cause mild to moderate respiratory distress, similar to rhinovirus or "the common cold[7,18]." In actuality, about 40-50% of common cold symptoms are caused by rhinoviruses and 15% by coronaviruses. Most people get infected with a coronavirus at some point of their lives.

The word "corona" comes from the Latin word for crown, and the virus was so named for the viruses' crown like projections. Coronaviruses were first discovered in the 1930s in North Dakota chickens. The new born chicks suffered from gasping and listlessness and a mortality rate between 40 and 90%. The

Common Coronavirus Symptoms:
- Runny nose
- Sore throat
- Headache
- Fever
- Cough
- Malaise (feeling unwell)

Complications (usually occur in patients with immune compromise or comorbidities):
- Pneumonia
- Bronchitis
- ARDS (acute respiratory distress syndrome)

virus was first isolated in humans in the 1960s. Over the past 20 years there have been three extremely severe strains of coronavirus in humans, including the most lethal of all—COVID-19.

Most coronaviruses infect bats, pigs, camels, and cats, causing enteritis (inflammation of the intestines) and respiratory symptoms[13,17]. Some, like COVID-19, "spilled over" to humans. In 2012, MERS, a coronavirus strain that transmitted from camels to humans, caused fatalities in the Middle East. This strain still causes minor outbreaks. In 2019, the SARS-CoV2 virus known as COVID-19 emerged. It shares 80% sequence identity with SARS-CoV1[20] but has already been far more lethal. COVID-19 is the first coronavirus in history to be declared a pandemic.

No vaccines or antivirals have been FDA approved to treat coronaviruses, but numerous human trials for both are currently being conducted.

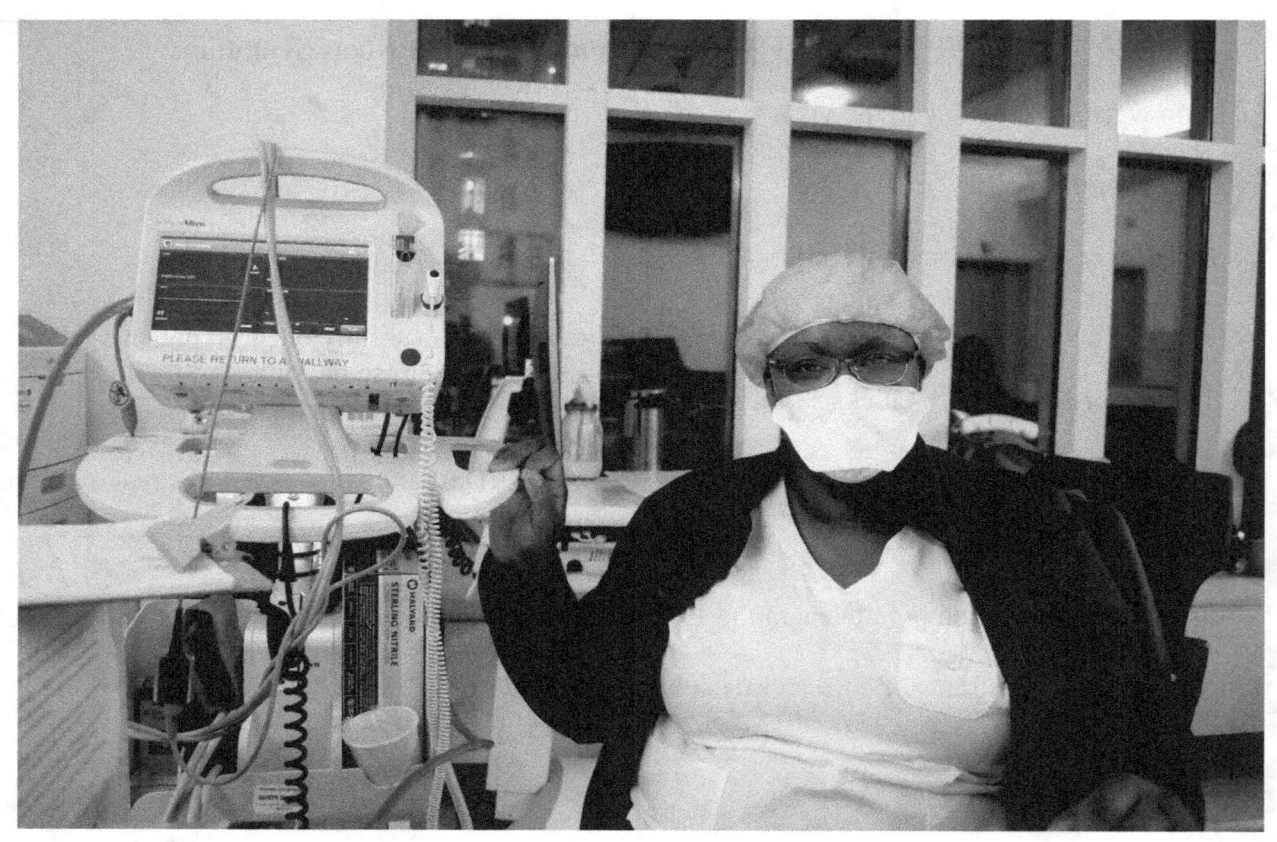

"Mission accepted."

-Michelle Trew-Palmer, Registered Nurse, Emergency Department, NYC

Underreported Disability

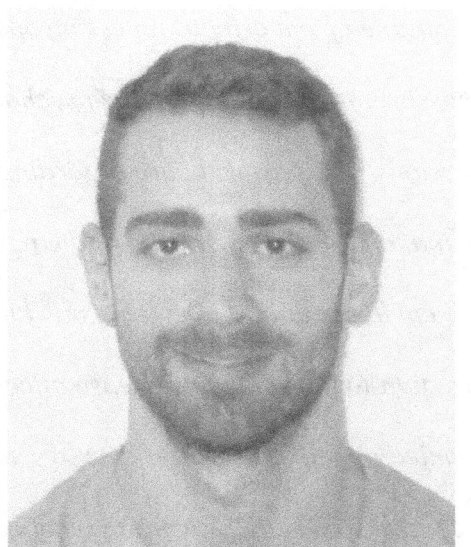

-Lorenzo Casertano, Physical Therapist, NYC

What was it like to work as a physical therapist at the peak of the pandemic? *At the beginning of the pandemic, we weren't sure what our role would be, but as it went on, it became very stressful. I felt we were one of the few people spending significant time with the patients, who were very lonely. Psychiatry and pastoral care were providing care through iPads, and I appreciate their efforts, but for some patients that wasn't enough. Although we are not trained in mental health counseling, we provide companionship and support during this difficult time.*

How did your role as a physical therapist change? *I am neurologically specialized, but during the pandemic I did more ICU level care with a lot of cardiopulmonary patients. We had a crash course in oxygen titration and management. Patients were more medically unstable than we are used to. There were also patients with strokes and neurological sequela such as peripheral nerve injuries. We are doing some case studies on these patients.*

What would you like people to know about COVID-19? *My wife brought up something that has stuck with me—we talk a lot about the death toll from the disease, but not about the severe and prolonged disability in the survivors. They don't report the numbers of kidney injury, liver damage, strokes, peripheral nerve injuries, or those who remain severely* *debilitated from critical illness myopathy. This is a huge deal and disability has taken a massive toll. There is also the psychological impact on healthcare workers. We had multiple sessions with pastoral care regarding staff nervousness about being infected, the constant grind, and the political side of the pandemic. My wife didn't want me to treat COVID patients if I could avoid it. I knew that my daughter is less at risk but my wife is pregnant and early on we didn't know how the disease affected pregnant women. I am in a leadership role and wanted to help, but was of course scared to bring it home. I took a few tests which came back negative so our PPE seems to be effective. I literally had patients giving me hugs. I was gowning, wearing N95 masks, and had boots on top of that. Every day I would take off my scrubs before coming to work and shower once I got home. One of my wife's friends died, and she was only 30 years old. This was shocking and made me realize that I am not immune. We see the worst of the worst and we know what can happen.*

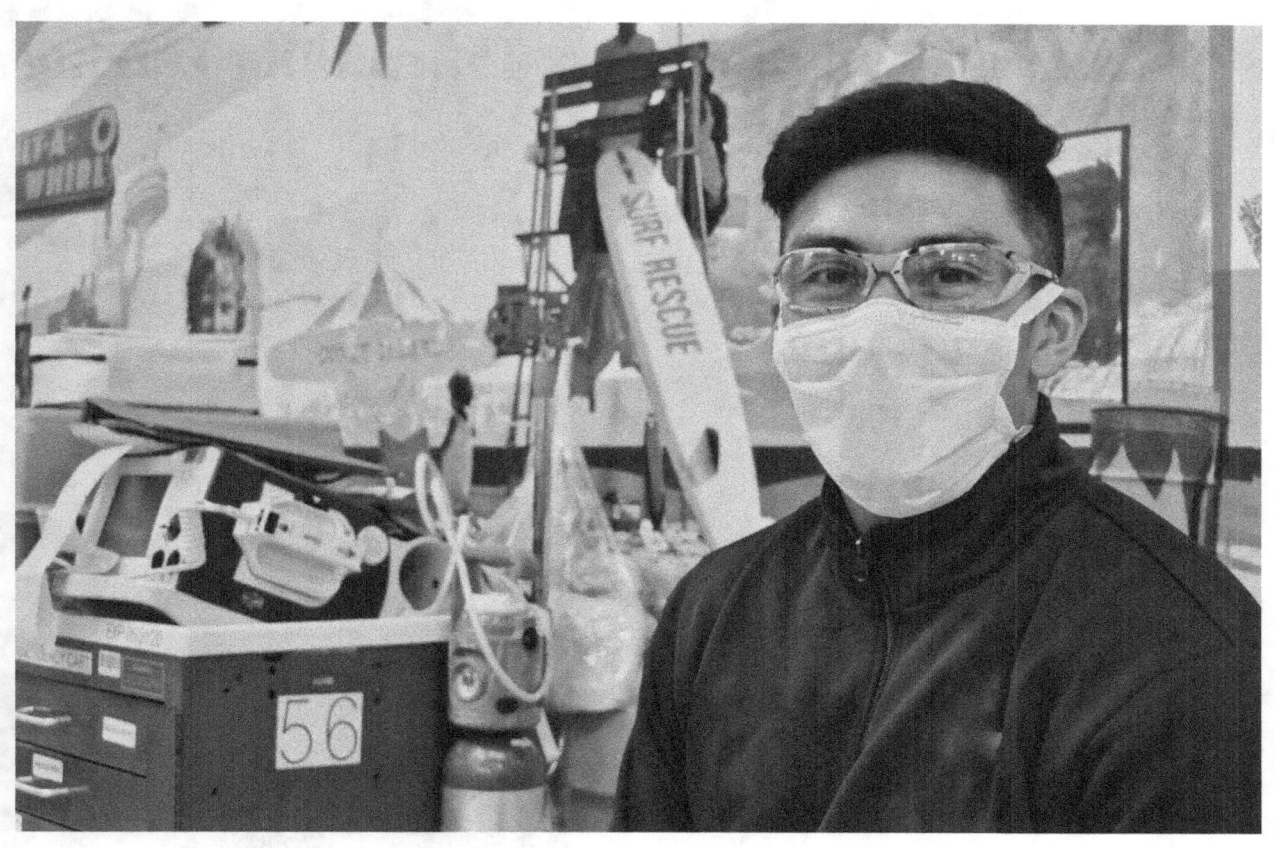

"I'm an asthmatic. My mother, brother, and father are all asthmatics. I know all too well the painful feeling of grasping for air. I see myself and my family in a lot of these patients who all of a sudden can't breathe because of this disease. I want to ease that weight on their chests.

-Paul Luardo, Registered Nurse, Emergency Department, NYC

Stream of Consciousness Journaling During Redeployment to the Emergency Department

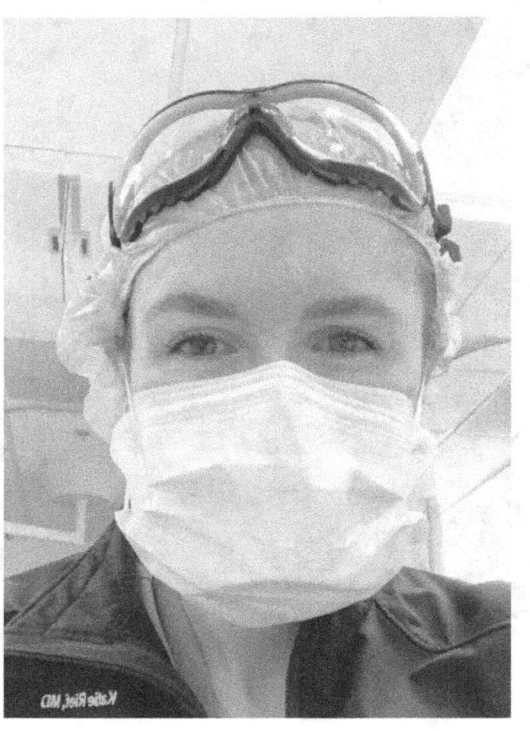

—Dr. Katie Rief, MD, Physical Medicine & Rehabilitation Resident Physician, NYC

Day 50 something? I haven't been counting. I had to look it up, from the first day we got the hint things were really wrong...March 3rd, 68 days ago. That was the day all domestic travel to conferences was banned. By the next week, our first ever Chief Resident meeting, March 10th, was the first and last time I've been in the same room with our leadership team. Following March 10th, we made the decision to suspend in-person didactics. HSS (Hospital for Special Surgery, one of our program's affiliates) shifted to all remote learning as well. And then on March 18th, HSS suspended all outpatient clinics and elective surgeries.

Programs scrambled to redeploy doctors and nurses, reorganize staff and expand ICU capacity. The hospital system expanded ICU bed capacity from 422 to 970 in 19 days. Incredible.

I worked my first shift in the ER March 27th and continued there until mid-May.

Life in NYC shut down but thank God, I could still go to work.

PPE was scarce throughout, but in mid and late March, at critically low levels. Fear combined with poor health literacy meant much of our supply was wasted on people not in direct patient care roles. I wore the same N95 mask for a few shifts at a time. Nothing compared to hospitals where they wore them for a week or more. Products designed to be single use, one encounter. Compared to places like Elmhurst/Queens etc., we were in great shape. Columbia was hardest hit in mid to late March. As overwhelming as it was in some ways, it was also algorithmic.

What's the sat? <90: add nasal cannula (NC), no more than 6L b/c it could create more aerosolization. Still <90: add a nonrebreather (NRB). Once you are maxed out on 6L of NC and 10 of NRB, call the ICU, the patient will likely be intubated at some point. Utilize awake proning- essentially rolling people around until they tired out and need a definitive airway.

So much to process. I am thankful beyond belief, to be in it, to be helping, to be working, learning. I get to be in the ER, forever my favorite place in the hospital.

It is unnatural being stuck inside for so long. Disconnected from community. No circus, no gyms, no bars/restaurants. No happy hour, no sports. It rained all of April. Truly the cruelest month. Mental health has suffered dramatically, I care for so many more suicide attempts on shifts these days. Our own Dr. Lorna Breen, site director for the Allen Hospital took her own life last week.

I miss my family. I miss the people I love. Maybe I should be more concerned about getting the virus, but I'm not. In all likelihood, I would be miserable for a week and then recover.

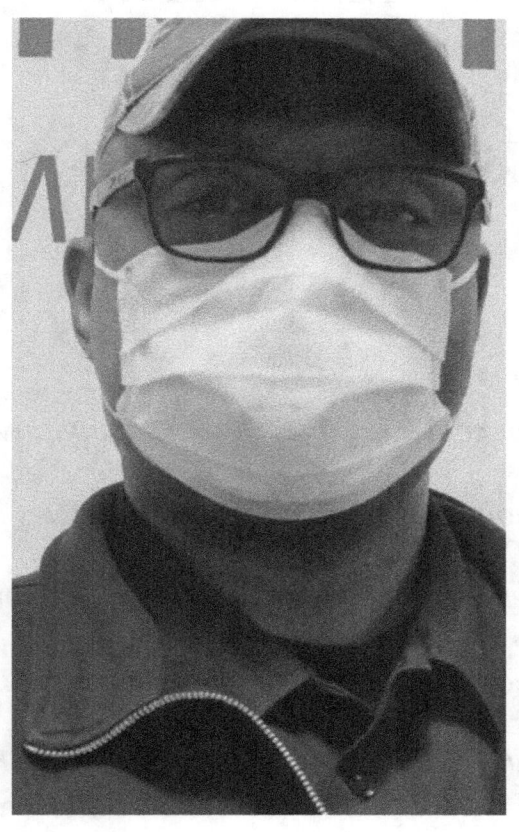

"Proud and happy to do this work, but frankly I'm scared. I am motivated by the people of NY, my family, friends, and my coworkers."

-Alexander Massac, Paramedic, NYC

CHAPTER 4:

PATHOLOGY OF COVID-19

"Pandemics often come in waves and the cumulative "morbidity" rate- the number of people who get sick in all the waves combined- often exceeds 50 percent. One virologist considers influenza so infectious that he calls it "a special instance" among infectious diseases, "transmitted so effectively that it exhausts the supply of susceptible hosts.""

-John M. Barry in *The Great Influenza*

The pathological findings of COVID-19 greatly resemble that of acute respiratory distress syndrome (ARDS),[10] which is a life-threatening complication that can arise from influenza, pneumonia, and pulmonary edema[39]. ARDS develops in 40% of COVID-19 patients and 50% of those who develop ARDS eventually die. Despite the terrifying lethality of the disease in the most severe cases, most cases of COVID-19 are asymptomatic or mild. This poses risk of transmission through asymptomatic carriers.

The CoV genome encodes 4 main structural proteins- the spike, envelope, membrane, and nucleocapsid proteins[16]. Similar to other SARS-CoV, COVID-19 uses the entry receptor

ACE2. Treatment with anti-ACE2 antibodies has been shown to disrupt binding of the virus to the receptor[13]; thus, manufacture of antibodies that bind to this receptor is being investigated as a potential COVID-19 treatment. ACE-2 has homology to ACE, which is a key enzyme in the renin-angiotensin system that is targeted in hypertension[21]. If you take an ACE-inhibitor (losartan, valsartan) for hypertension, your blood pressure is lowered through inhibition of this system. ACE-2 is expressed in the lungs, kidney, and GI tract—explaining why COVID-19 affects these organs.

Mortality from COVID-19 was initially estimated to be 2.5%, but appears to be closer to 0.2 to 0.6%[30]. The death rate in the United States is 1.3%.[108] This differs from the case fatality rate, which compares the number of deaths to the number of people diagnosed, rather than the entire population. The case fatality rate will be highest when countries are experiencing a peak in cases.

> **What is the case fatality rate?**
>
> It measures the number of deaths per patient diagnosed with a disease. This differs from the mortality rate, which estimates the percent of the population that dies from the disease.

COVID-19 predominantly affects elderly patients with comorbidities such as obesity, hypertension (HTN), diabetes mellitus (DM), and cancer. Ninety-five percent of patients who have died from the disease had such comorbidities. COVID-19 first affects the body through direct injury, but one of the most dangerous parts of the infection is a hyper-inflammatory state due to an overproduction of cytokines. We use the inflammatory marker C-reactive protein (CRP) to measure patients' levels of acute inflammation and to monitor their disease severity.

Lymphopenia, a reduction in lymphocytes, is also a very common finding in COVID-19 patients. At the peak of the disease, swabs were a scarce commodity and had to be rationed for the most likely cases. Lymphopenia, elevated CRP levels, and chest x-ray findings of bilateral patchy infiltrates were used in conjunction with patients' signs and symptoms to determine who warranted testing. Now as swabs have become more available at the three hospitals where I worked, all hospitalized patients and staff are tested, sometimes on multiple occasions.

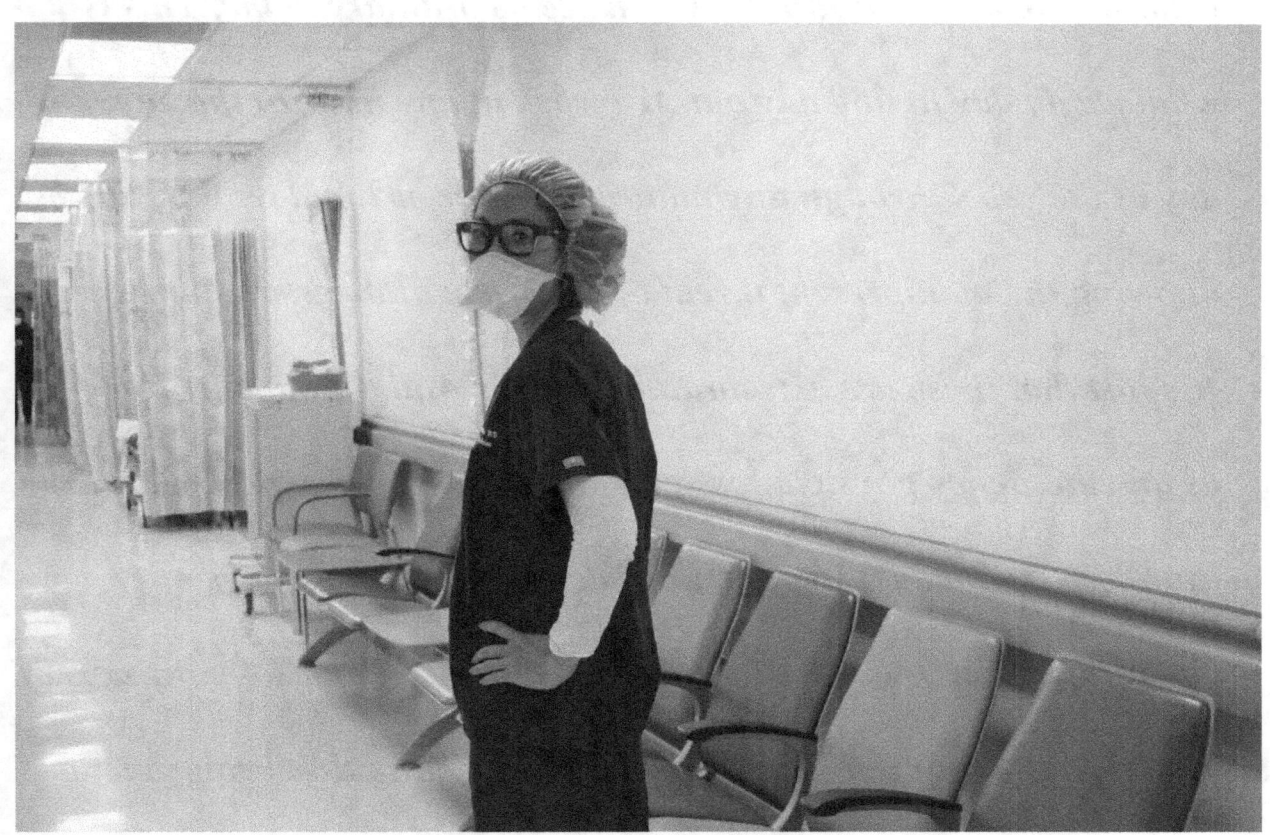

"There is something absolutely beautiful about working during a pandemic: a true emergency, an event of great need with epic consequences. It is the greatest honor to have the training and education to serve in this capacity. There is a phenomenal team atmosphere among all emergency department staff and consultants. We're tirelessly researching and collaborating with peers to try to understand a new and dynamic disease in order to save our city. There is a stronger connection to our patients: I see the fear in their eyes and it's the same fear I see when I look in the mirror. Many see

what we do as extraordinary. But it seems ordinary to me. This is what we do day in and day out. We work at any hour of the day, any day of the year, through any natural disaster or holiday. We work knowing the omnipresent threat of terrorism and personal injury. It's just that these are extraordinary times. And the support I've felt as an emergency physician is something I've never experienced. The thunderous applause at 7pm, the sidewalk chalk messages of encouragement, the donations of food and PPE, and so many acts of kindness and love…it's an overwhelming feeling that brings me to tears every time. When the pandemic dies down, I will be thrilled to hug my family and friends, dine in a restaurant, take a trip, and do all the things that I took for granted. But I will also look back with great fondness for this storm- even though it will probably bring indescribable pain and loss- because we weathered it together.

-Dr. Lindsey Kurumada, MD, Emergency Room Attending Physician, NYC

Caring for Adults with Severe Mental Illness

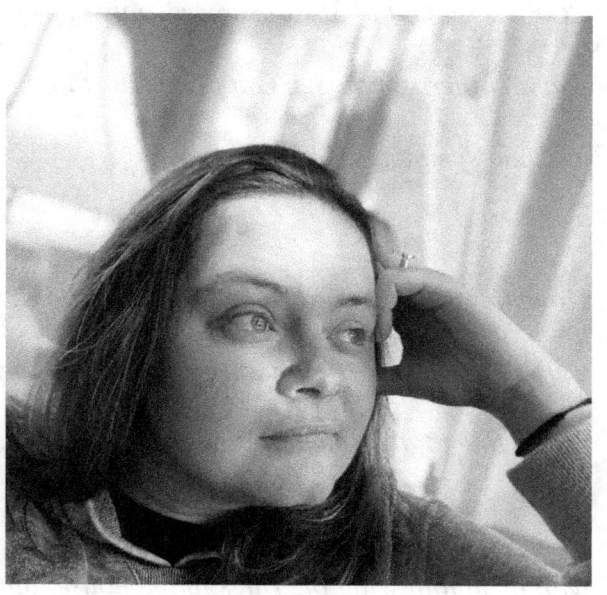

- *Catherine Migel, Licensed Clinical Social Worker and Manager of Adult Group Homes*

What was it like to work in adult group homes during the pandemic? *It started out chaotic and scary. There were a lot of unknowns and no precedent on how to handle them. There was also the issue of accessing supplies (cleaning and food). We were left to get these items on our own and it was often really difficult to track things down, especially disinfectant and antibacterial items. The consumers were essentially quarantined in their homes. Most of them did not understand what was going on or the severity of the issue. As the pandemic went on, though, things calmed down and we managed everything better. The most difficult aspect was the staffing. Two of the homes I manage have to be staffed 24/7 and a lot of the staff have medical conditions themselves, or had to balance childcare, so making sure all of the houses were appropriately staffed was a challenge throughout the last few months.*

Did any of your patients contract the disease? Thankfully none of the consumers contracted COVID-19. Out of 38 consumers, only one spiked a fever but it passed after a day and they had no other symptoms. Out of my 20 staff members, I was the only one who tested positive and had symptoms.

How did patients react to having no visitors? We had to do a lot of education regarding COVID-19 and why they were not allowed to go out in public. Often times we had to repeat things due to their mental illnesses. It was helpful when they would hear about things on the news or their families would also tell them about the dangers. A lot of times we have issues with them following the rules in the house, but once they understood we didn't make up these rules, they seemed more compliant. We stopped all visits, which many consumers rely on. We had one consumer who became very depressed and symptomatic because he could no longer spend weekends with his mother.

What are some of the experiences that most affected you? Many of my consumers have co-occurring conditions (substance use, serious medical issues). Due to the pandemic, there were no in-person NA/AA meetings, and most of their medical appointments were cancelled or changed to virtual. We had to set up all of the houses to be able to access Zoom and other video teleconferencing services. Our consumers aren't exactly computer savvy so it was a big adjustment for them and our staff.

What would you like people to know about COVID-19? I know from personal experience contracting COVID-19 that it is a very isolating disease. I really understood how people were *saying that there was an increase in mental health issues during the pandemic, because I felt completely isolated during my whole quarantine. I also had a lot of anxiety regarding rejoining the public and being near anyone afterward.*

What was your personal experience getting COVID-19? *Thankfully I had very mild symptoms. One day I had a lot of nasal congestion. I usually get bad seasonal allergies, so I figured that was the cause. I was taking some cold medicine and still going into work but isolating myself from the clients and staff. I think a day or so after I started having nasal issues I was going to sleep one night and felt a little short of breath. I then woke up and looked into getting tested. That was probably a Thursday, and I got tested that Sunday. I stayed home from work until the results came back. They came back on a Wednesday and at that point I had lost all sense of taste and smell so I figured it would be positive. I live with my mother who has COPD so my biggest fear was that I gave it to her somehow. Thankfully she didn't exhibit any symptoms.*

Overall, it was just very isolating. I had previously worked in a group home for adults with HIV and it reminded me of our clients who spoke about how having HIV gave them feelings of loneliness, guilt, and shame. It was a weird, unexpected feeling that most COVID positive patients don't discuss. My doctor had me stay home for 2 weeks and I self-quarantined in my bedroom. When I returned to work I did have lingering symptoms of extreme exhaustion. It was really difficult for me to wake up or get out of bed for a few weeks.

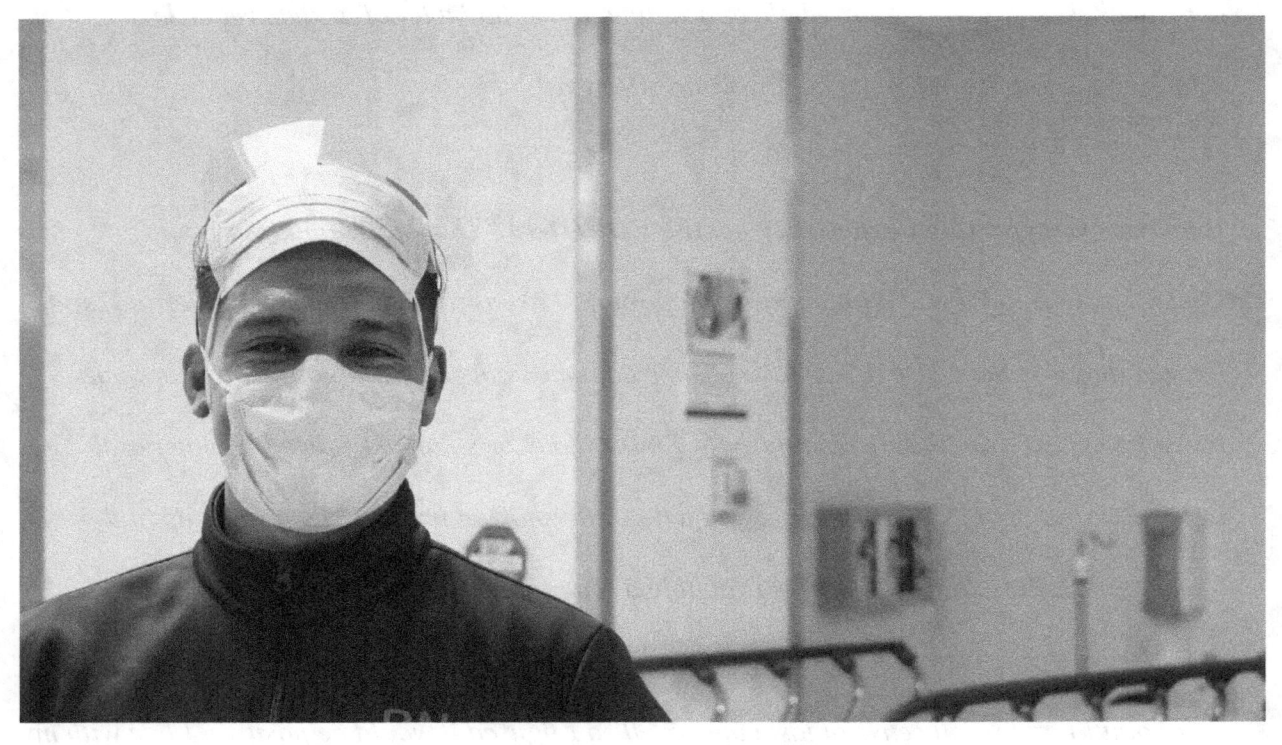

"I see the mountain we are up against but I also see the miracles headed our way."

- **Robert Serrano, Registered Nurse, Emergency Department, NYC**

CHAPTER 5:

INITIAL TRANSMISSION OF COVID-19

"For whatever was attacking these sailors was not only spreading, it was spreading explosively."

-John M. Barry in *The Great Influenza*

Phylogenetic analysis, a computational approach that evaluates the evolution of traits through DNA sequencing, has determined that the first cases of COVID-19 originated in Wuhan China sometime between October and December of 2019.

The novel coronavirus is thought to have been transmitted from bats given its 88% similarity to two bat-derived SARS-CoV strains[19]. From bats, it likely went to an intermediary wildlife host before reaching humans. While the exact location of human transmission is unclear, widespread explosion of the disease has been traced to the Huanan Seafood Wholesale Market of Wuhan, China. There has been speculation that the virus was developed in a laboratory in China but there is no evidence to support this theory.

The index case, patient zero, first exhibited symptoms on December 1st, 2019[9]. He was a man in his 70s with Alzheimer's disease who lived several bus rides away from the Wuhan seafood market and did not leave his home. Multiple cases of pneumonia must have sprouted this month, but the novel coronavirus would not be discovered and/or reported until the end of the month. On December 24th, a bronchoalveolar lavage (BAL) sample was sent for a patient with continued respiratory symptoms despite typical care. Three days later this sample returned positive for a novel coronavirus and the patient was quarantined. Over the next few days more patients who had been exposed to the Wuhan seafood market were found to have similar respiratory symptoms and a December 30th lab test report claimed the occurrence of SARS. The Wuhan Municipal Health Commission made a public announcement to the city of a pneumonia outbreak and the first international report was released. The US CDC first learned of the 27 cases of pneumonia in Wuhan on December 31st, but as per the South China Morning Post, Chinese authorities had identified 266 people who had been infected at this time. The disease was referred to as 2019-nCoV, later named COVID-19[28].

How is COVID-19 transmitted?

COVID-19 is transmitted through droplets and thus masks and disinfectants can help to disrupt its spread. In May, the CDC released findings that COVID-19 is much more easily transmitted from person to person than via contact with contaminated surfaces.

For how long can people transmit the virus?[114]

Recent evidence shows that virus shedding decreases as symptoms resolve. That being said, it is still unknown for how long people may shed the virus. Currently, it recommended for those who are infected to self-quarantine for 10 days from onset of illness and 3 days after recovery, as transmission rate after this time approaches zero.

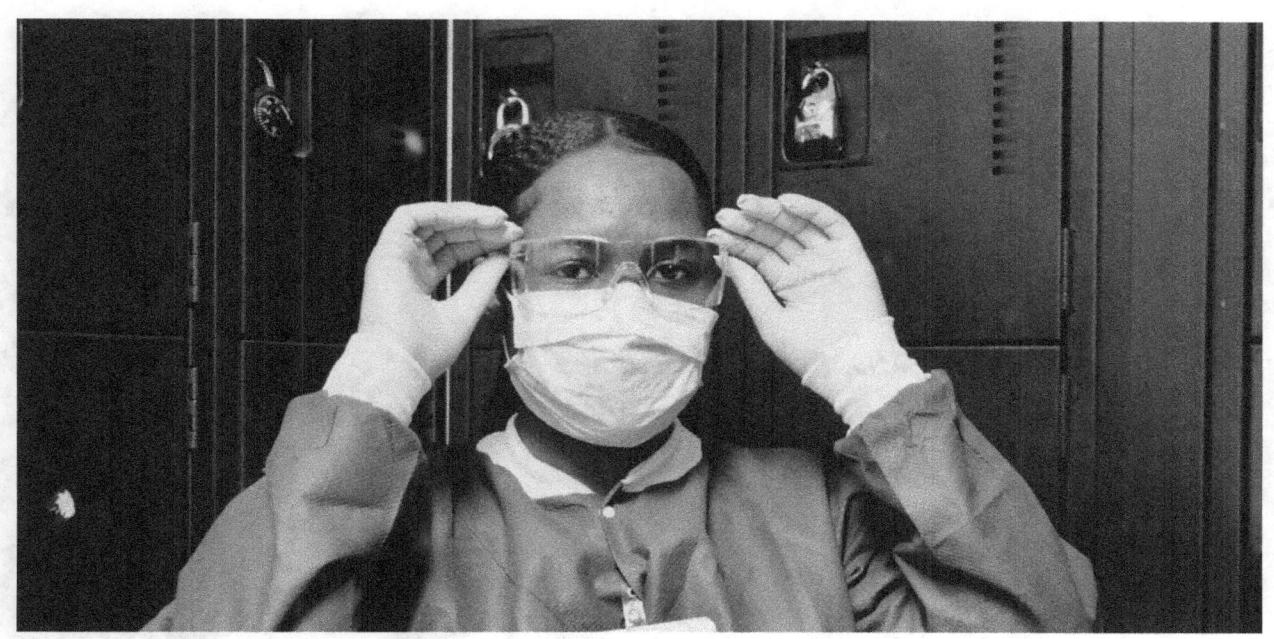

"This is very stressful mentally, physically, and emotionally for patients and for myself. Through this experience I learned that my coworkers are more like family the way we hold each other down helping us to push through the shift together as a unit."

-**Gerlene Valcin, Registered Nurse, Emergency Department, NYC**

Redeployed to the Surgical ICU (SICU)

—Dr. Vera Tsetlina, MD, Physical Medicine & Rehabilitation Resident Physician, NYC

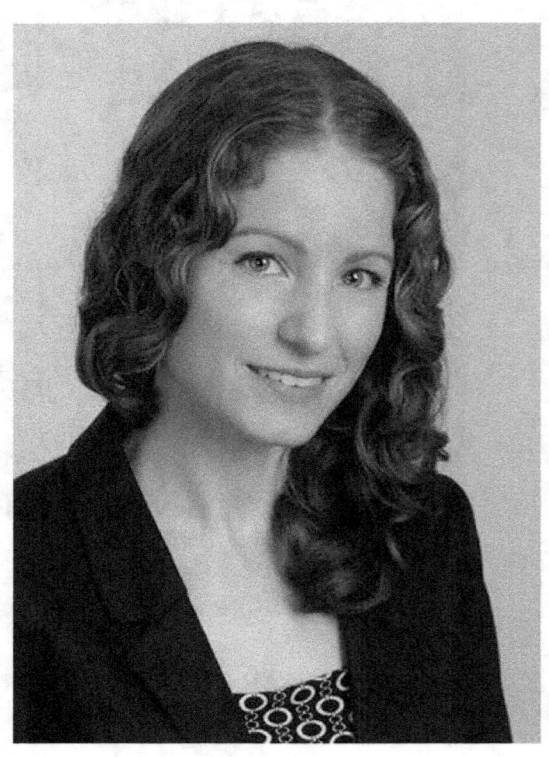

What was it like to be redeployed in the SICU? It was actually a very interesting, rewarding, and meaningful experience for me.

How was the SICU reorganized to cope with COVID? Pre-COVID, the SICU was staffed by anesthesiology. Because of COVID, all the anesthesia attendings, residents and fellows were working in the ICU ORs. SICU was led by interventional cardiology attendings, which was hard for them because running an ICU team is not something they usually do. Medicine ICU attendings were there to advice on ventilator management and other issues.

Below each cardiology attending was a cardiology fellow, and below the fellow was someone like me. My role was called "First call". We were the ones putting in all the orders and checking labs, the ones who called families with updates, the ones who would be called for any change in the patient's condition. We knew everything about our patients and worked closely with nurses to resolve any issues that came up. This role is usually filled by a resident. In our case it was residents and doctors from all over the hospital: I had a pediatric *endocrinology attending working next to me every day, psychiatry residents, three pediatric hematology-oncology attendings and pediatric fellows. Each of us faced different challenges. For example, pediatric physicians had been to the ICU multiple times in their training, but they have never managed adult patients and medication dosing is completely different. Therefore, it was big adjustment, but they handled it admirably.*

Who spends the most time with patients? *Nurses do. Surgical ICU nurses are outstanding. I have never seen nurses so well-trained, thoughtful, and knowledgeable. They enjoy what they do, and they have amazing personalities. They are true heroes and I can't say enough about them.*

Was there high rate of burnout? *There was definitely burnout. Different departments were redeploying physicians to the SICU and each had a different policy. I was the only person from rehab. There were always 2-3 people from psych. Psychiatry residents have amazing qualities which allowed them to learn, perform, and cope. None had any prior exposure to the ICU, whereas I had at least 3 months in my residency training. I still remember my first day in the ICU vividly, and their first days were in the COVID unit! The second week is much better than the first as you learn your patients and the SICU flow. The third and fourth weeks became more difficult and that's when burnout was highest.*

Were staff infected? *By the time I started my redeployment (it was right before the peak) our unit had plenty of PPE. None of the people whom I worked with got sick or tested positive* with PCR swabs. We were very conscientious about wearing PPE properly. My colleague called me "the queen of donning and doffing!"

Was it difficult that family members could not visit? In the beginning, it was very challenging because we had to learn to talk to the families so they could feel what was going on with their loved ones and so they could make informed decisions about their care. We used Facetime and different video applications. Our hospital allowed these to be used because they were so beneficial to the patients. I would show them what the patients' rooms were like, I would point to different tubes and explain the rationale for each. We were able to get iPads to leave inside the patients' rooms so that patients could spend time with their families. It was such an enlightening experience to see how patients wake up to the sound of their family members voices.

One of the attendings told me that on other units, nurses and staff would put a short bio about the patients on their doors so we would know something other than weight/height and vitals. I started to ask my patients' family members about different things in their lives--what did they like to eat, what did they like to do in their spare time. It was wonderful for the team to know something about our patients' personal lives.

What things did you do relieve stress during the pandemic? Ballet, walking, biking, exploring the parts of the city to see how it looks during the pandemic. At first with no traffic and crowds, the city looked so beautiful. However, later on my husband and I realized that the city has lost its heart beat. The life of the city is the people. We started to miss it so much. And finally, it's started to come back.

I have to say that we received enormous amount of support from the community. We were getting all these cards and letters from kids all over the country. We were also getting food. The 7 pm clapping kept me going even on the hardest days. I'm very thankful for that.

What would you like people to know about COVID-19? *I would like people to see Covid-19 as I see it: if you follow precautions and be careful, it's possible to avoid getting sick. I worked with COVID patients in the ICU and now in rehab and did not get sick or have symptoms. I want people to protect themselves by avoiding unnecessary risks.*

Do you think antibody testing is accurate? *No.. If it is positive it does mean you have had COVID or possibly other coronaviruses. If it is negative it doesn't mean that you didn't have it.*

Final thoughts? *In life and in medicine and especially in this pandemic, you can always find someone who can answer your questions and help you get where you*

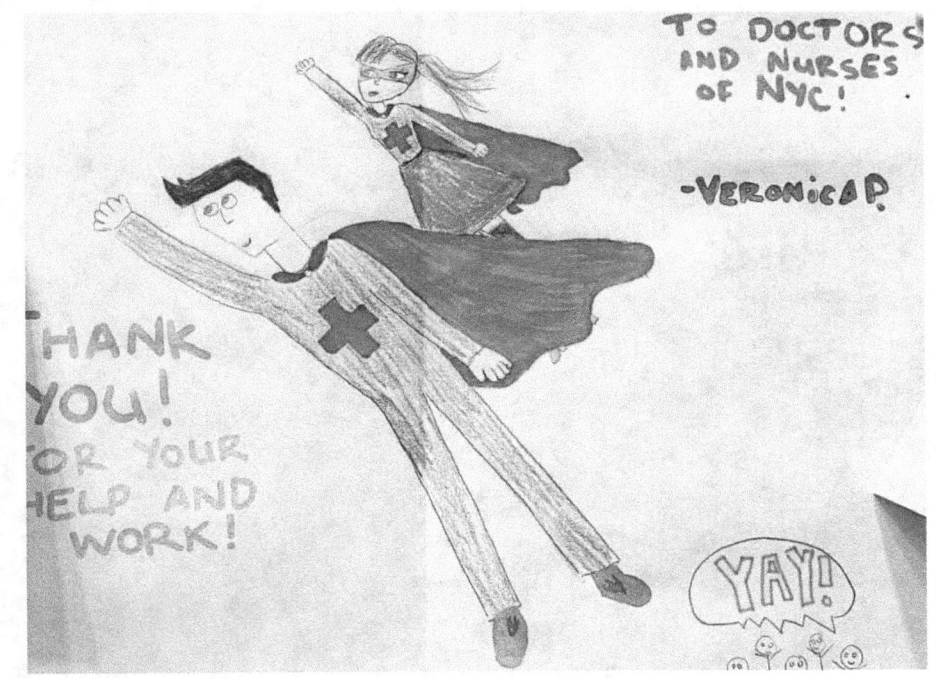

need to be. You need to pause to think what to ask and who to ask. We were not ICU physicians, but we were smart enough to ask questions. We all came from different medical backgrounds and our knowledge and sense of the world were so different. We were helping each other, and we were getting help. In the end, we had this sense of camaraderie. Together we were more than each of us as individuals. I am very, very grateful for the opportunity to be of help, and that I had the knowledge and skills to do so.

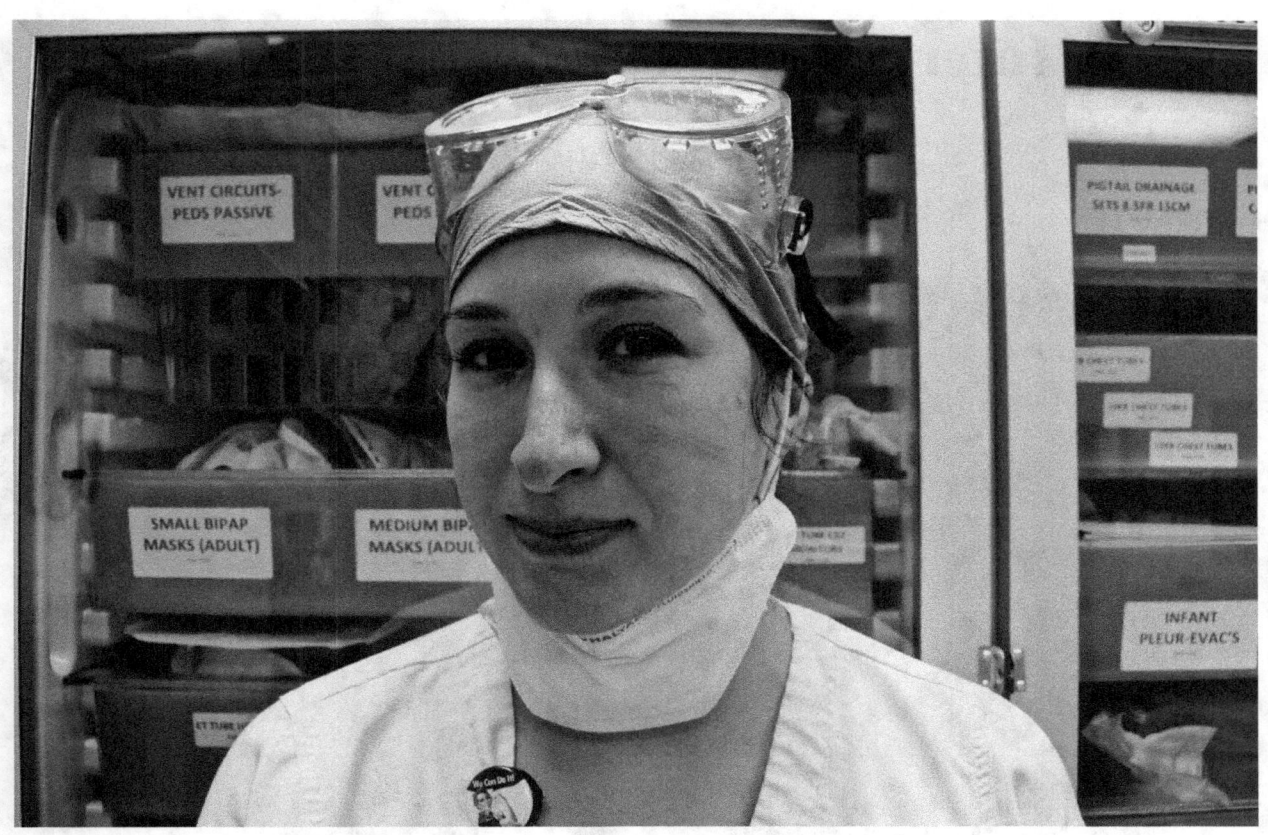

"I love the ER because I love saving lives. We see a lot of crazy and sometimes horrible things, but we also see miracles happen every day. Like when we code a person in cardiac arrest and suddenly get a pulse back. There is literally no better high than that. We get to bring people back to life…after they've died! It's the most amazing feeling. I think people can best support the frontlines by STAYING HOME and flattening this curve!"

-Jessica Trosterud, Registered Nurse, Emergency Department, NYC

International Perspective: India

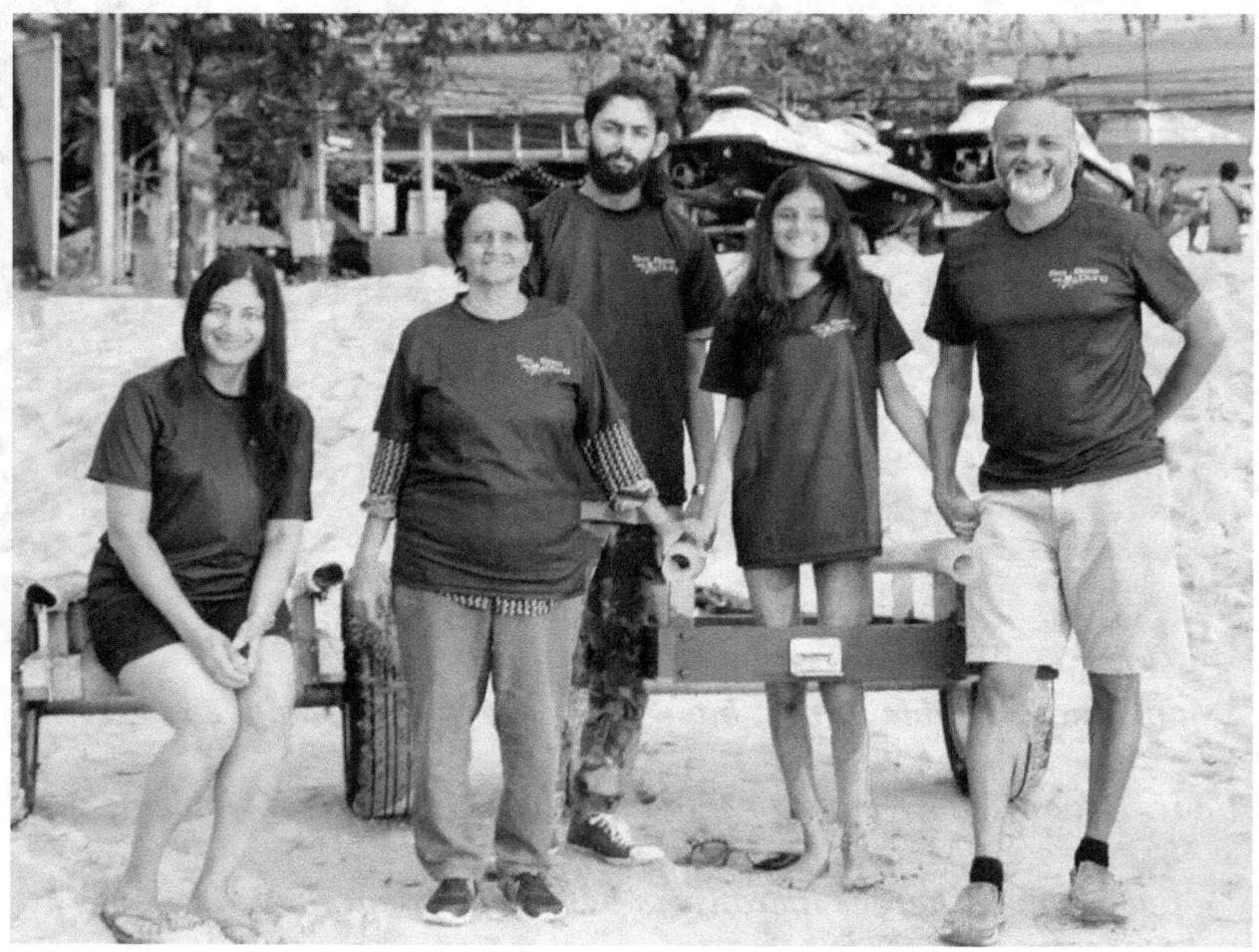

— *Anu and Sanjay Ganapathy, CEO of SPAN Healthcare*

How has the pandemic affected you personally? *Our perspective is skewed in the sense that while social interactions and travel are curtailed, we live in a relative "golden-cage" of safety and support. So, yes, we have the need to plan purchases, quarantine goods (including perishables) outside the home for 24 hours, wash as many of the products as possible etc., but our lives for most part is comfortable. We can certainly imagine how different it would be for* *folks who are daily wage workers – and there are a lot of them. We were primarily concerned for our mothers, both of whom are older and at higher risk – but they have been quite well and resilient.*

How has the lockdown affected your community? *Initially in India this was mostly a rich-person's disease, since the virus passed into our country through international travelers. Curtailing the contact between them and the masses was the goal of the first lockdown which was initiated on March 23, 2020 when the number of infected individuals numbered less than 500. This lockdown was initially slated to end on April 14, 2020 but was subsequently extended until May 3, 2020. Its goal was the following:*

1. *Prevention and/or delay of community-level transmissions*

2. *Flattening the curve and building treatment and care infrastructure targeting COVID 19*

3. *Building wider and secure testing capability*

By the time the lockdown ended, our key success in a country as large and populous as India was that EVERYONE knew about the existence of the virus. Most recognized also the dangers this disease posed in a densely populated country like India without the doctor: patient and patient: bed ratios available in advanced countries.

Another positive from the lockdown is that citizens have a greater appreciation for our local health administrators and police, who are generally reviled. Through contact tracing, road barricading, and home follow-ups, they have made a yeoman effort to keep the general populace safe, and I hope that this new-born respect will endure past COVID times!

Despite these positives, one negative is that India failed to accommodate the impact of the sudden lockdown on the labor that the cities rely on to run their industries, construction, restaurants, hotels, and other establishments. These millions were marginalized as their workplaces shut abruptly, denying them their source of livelihood, sustenance, and shelter—since a number of them sleep where they work. The state and federal governments were also flat-footed in terms of providing shelter, food, and water to these citizens. Towards the middle of April when the lockdown was extended to May 3rd, one of the largest and most unfortunate journeys in our nation was triggered - with millions streaming home hundreds of miles away, on foot and otherwise. This caused untold and documented misery that will remain an enduring image of the failure of the government to provide to its neediest citizens.

The governments also failed to build the necessary infrastructure during the lockdown. This was a particularly conflicted time with reports that suggested India may have been provided with quasi-divine intervention due to the following:

- *the relatively high temperatures*

- *higher levels of immunity inherent among Indians due to exposure to infections*

- *post-natal and juvenile inoculation regimens that may have provided added protection*

- *what seemed like very low mortality rates*

How has SPAN Healthcare been affected? *The Indian economy was already under severe pressure on account of governmental policies which, while contemplated with the appropriate objectives and intentions, had depressed the trajectory of growth. The lockdown seriously exacerbated the impact. The entrepreneurial spirit that underpinned decades of growth has been critically impaired, and with long-term consequences.*

The industry of which we are part– provision of equipment and disposables to blood banks, hematologists and the laboratory services we run—was severely impacted because of the following factors:

1. *The large corporate organizations which provided a significant percentage of voluntary blood were effectively shut*

2. *Donors were subject to questioning when they volunteered to travel to donate blood on account of police personnel not adequately informed of the continued need for blood to run hospitals*

3. *Mobile camps at schools, apartment blocks, and religious organizations, were curtailed on account of the need for maintaining social distance*

4. *Curtailed movement meant lower sample loads at laboratories, and delayed treatment to the non-COVID patients who were not always free to move around*

5. *Lastly, hospitals, private and public, were required to set aside beds for the deluge of patients that were inevitable – but for a long time, most of these beds remained empty since the patients did not turn up in the numbers expected (this has now changed) and caused the hospitals to absorb large losses – driven by empty beds and a reluctance among the non-COVID patients to present at the hospitals which also accepted COVID patients*

So, we have had to trim our workforce by about 15%, a lot of the staff have taken pay-cuts ranging from 5 – 50% so that most of us are able to keep our jobs and benefits. However, the longer this goes on, the greater the likelihood of additional cuts.

SPAN has been involved in the collection of plasma for fractionation into albumin, immunoglobulins and factors. We were, therefore, uniquely positioned to assist with the treatment of intubated, end-state patients with antibodies collected from patients who had recovered from COVID 19. The treatment protocol set by the Indian regulatory authority, the ICMR, has been mostly found to be beneficial.

What was it like for your family when Nikhil was quarantined in South Africa? *Our son, Nikhil, went to South Africa to work at an environment protection program close to Cape Town. Two months into his job, South Africa imposed a lock down as well and he was compelled to stay with a most wonderful, generous family. They would pamper him in a beautiful home. While we were never worried about his safety there, we wanted to bring him back as soon as possible. There were repatriation flights out of South Africa bound for India and it was with a lot of assistance from friends, family and the Indian High Commission in South Africa, that he was able to come home. After a week of solitary quarantine in Hyderabad, he returned home for another week of confinement at home. He is 20-year-old healthy man and we were not worried for his health.*

What kind of interventions have the government used to protect the economy? *The government has tried to use legacy social security systems to reach the people most affected by this crisis, those living at or below the poverty line. However, in the current situation with so many upheavals, it has been difficult to identify and reach the correct beneficiary. The government initially promulgated labor protection laws that were, at the least, ill-conceived and, at worst, untenable and impossible to implement. As the disease unraveled and impact grew, it also became more and more obvious that there was little the government could do to balance the twin challenges of the growing disease and the sinking economy. It has finally chosen the former, and consequently, we gyrate between lockdowns and bouts of freedom.*

The fiscal support projected by the government was insubstantial, and even misleading, in the context of the size of the problem—but this is not just macro-economics—there are layers of micro-economic issues that must be anticipated. It has been a herculean task for any government, especially with the uncertainty of how long this pandemic will persist. Further fiscal support will necessarily include printing currency, which will further devalue the falling Indian Rupee and result in massive inflation—even stagflation if the factors of production are not restored.

Anything else you would like to add? *Everyone is appreciating time with family a lot more now. We were caught up in the rat race. Everyone has realized that we don't need to dress up and go out and party, or spend money unnecessarily. This has brought families together and calmed everyone down. It has done wonders for the environment. We have never seen such blue skies in Bangalore. India is usually so polluted. We have been able to hear the birds rather than the traffic. We have never seen anything like it before. Things happen for a reason and we just have to do our best. Even just picking up the phone and calling someone and asking if they need anything goes a long way. Depression and anxiety are rampant, people are not getting enough exercise. I know counselors who are providing free sessions due to increased mental health needs at this time. Attitude and resiliency are so important to deal with any disturbance in life. Never take anything for granted.*

CHAPTER 6:

COMPARISON TO PREVIOUS PANDEMICS

"Normally influenza chiefly kills the elderly and infants, but in the 1918 pandemic roughly half of those who died were young men and women in the prime of their life, in their twenties and thirties. Harvey Cushing, then a brilliant young surgeon who would go on to great fame- and who himself fell desperately ill with influenza and never recovered from what was likely a complication- would call these victims 'doubly dead in that they died so young'."

-John M. Barry in *The Great Influenza*

In 1665, the bubonic plaque killed more than a quarter of London's population and devastated Europe. Since "the Black Death," numerous pandemics have killed humans and created worldwide panic. How does COVID-19 compare?

The 1918 influenza pandemic

When I was an undergrad at Brown University, I was assigned to read John Barry's *The Great Influenza* for one of my classes. I couldn't put it down. If you haven't read this book, I would highly recommend it for a readable medical and social history of the 1918 influenza epidemic. After COVID-19 struck, I reread the book and found it all the more fascinating having been through medical school and caring for patients in the current pandemic. In 2018, John Barry added an afterword that is incredibly insightful regarding the challenges we would face in a future pandemic. I'm sure when he wrote this he didn't expect that COVID-19 was just two years away, but his theories regarding the virus's impact and the world's response have been remarkably accurate.

The 1918 pandemic, dubbed the Spanish Flu, is the most severe pandemic in the past century, affecting one-third of the world's population at the time[85]. This virulent and novel strain of influenza affected 500 million people worldwide, killing 50 million,[30] before it gradually faded away in 1920. Caused by an H1N1 virus and transmitted via birds, it was known as the Spanish Flu due to its media coverage in Spain—a neutral country in the first World War, and one of the few countries to report accurately on the magnitude of the disease at that time[85]. Though recent studies suggest it originated in New York[85], its site of origin remains unknown. The Spanish Flu case fatality rate is estimated at 2%, which is currently higher than the COVID-19 case fatality rate, which is estimated to be between 0.2 and 0.6%. Unlike COVID-19, children were also highly susceptible to the Spanish Flu, and the most affected population were young adults between the ages of 20 and 40[85]. If COVID-19 were killing our children and young adults at such high rates, I imagine fear of the virus and adherence to social distancing would be much different.

The second wave of the Spanish Flu struck in the fall and was much deadlier than the first. It is thought that the virus may have mutated and possibly re-assorted into a more virulent strain. Those who were infected during the first wave were relatively protected from the more lethal second wave, during which the majority of deaths occurred. Pandemics characteristically wax and wane in multiple waves as viruses mutate and spread to different populations. This is why experts today warn that a resurgence of COVID-19 is likely, and some say "inevitable."

Swine Flu[115]

In the spring of 2009, a novel influenza virus known as the Swine Flu (H1N1) originated in the United States[115] and spread rapidly around the world, killing 575,400 people in the first year alone. 12,469 of these deaths were in the United States. In contrast to COVID-19, 80% of deaths were in people less than 65 years of age[30]. Nearly one-third of the population over age 60 had antibodies against the virus, likely due to prior exposure an H1N1 strain[115]. Flu vaccination offered little protection since this strain was so different from most other strains of flu. A vaccine was unavailable until after the peak of the virus had passed, similar to what we ae experiencing with COVID-19.

SARS-CoV1

When I heard mention of coronavirus in the news in early February, I didn't think much of it. We learned about coronaviruses in medical school, and few strains have had the morbidity and mortality caused by influenza each year. The most lethal coronavirus strain thus far was Severe Acute Respiratory Syndrome (SARS), which first emerged in the Guangdong province of southern China in November of 2002[13]. I was 12 years old at the time and was peripherally aware of this dangerous virus, which disappeared in 2004 after spreading through 29 countries and killing 774 people[13]. COVID-19 is more transmissible than SARS-CoV1, but the latter was deadlier, killing 10% of those infected[46]. SARS-CoV1 was controlled within 8 months, but experts feel COVID-19 will not be as easily contained. One reason is that unlike SARS-CoV1, COVID-19 patients appear to be infectious 1-2 days before first showing symptoms. This makes it more difficult to isolate infected patients and

---

What is the difference between a pandemic and an epidemic?

A pandemic describes when an epidemic is rampant through multiple countries; it is of a much greater magnitude. In Greek, "pan" means "all," and "demos" means "people."[46] It is defined by how widespread an infection is, rather than how many people it has killed[46]. Experts use the term pandemic to signal that attempts to contain the virus have failed and that there must be greater concerted effort to combat the disease and to prepare hospitals for an influx of patients[46].

---

perform thorough contact tracing.

How does COVID-19 compare to the regular flu?

For the 2019 flu season, the Center for Disease Control (CDC) estimates that there were between 39,000,000 and 56,000,000 cases and 24,000 to 62,000 deaths in the United States alone[6]. COVID-19 shares some similarities to the flu: they are both viruses that primarily affect the respiratory tract and are most severe in people older than 65. However,

COVID-19 is more infectious and causes more hospitalizations and deaths than influenza[52]. The COVID-19 case fatality rate is estimated to be about 10 times that of the flu during a typical season[85]. And unlike the flu, we have no vaccine for COVID-19 so it is likely to infect a much larger portion of the population.

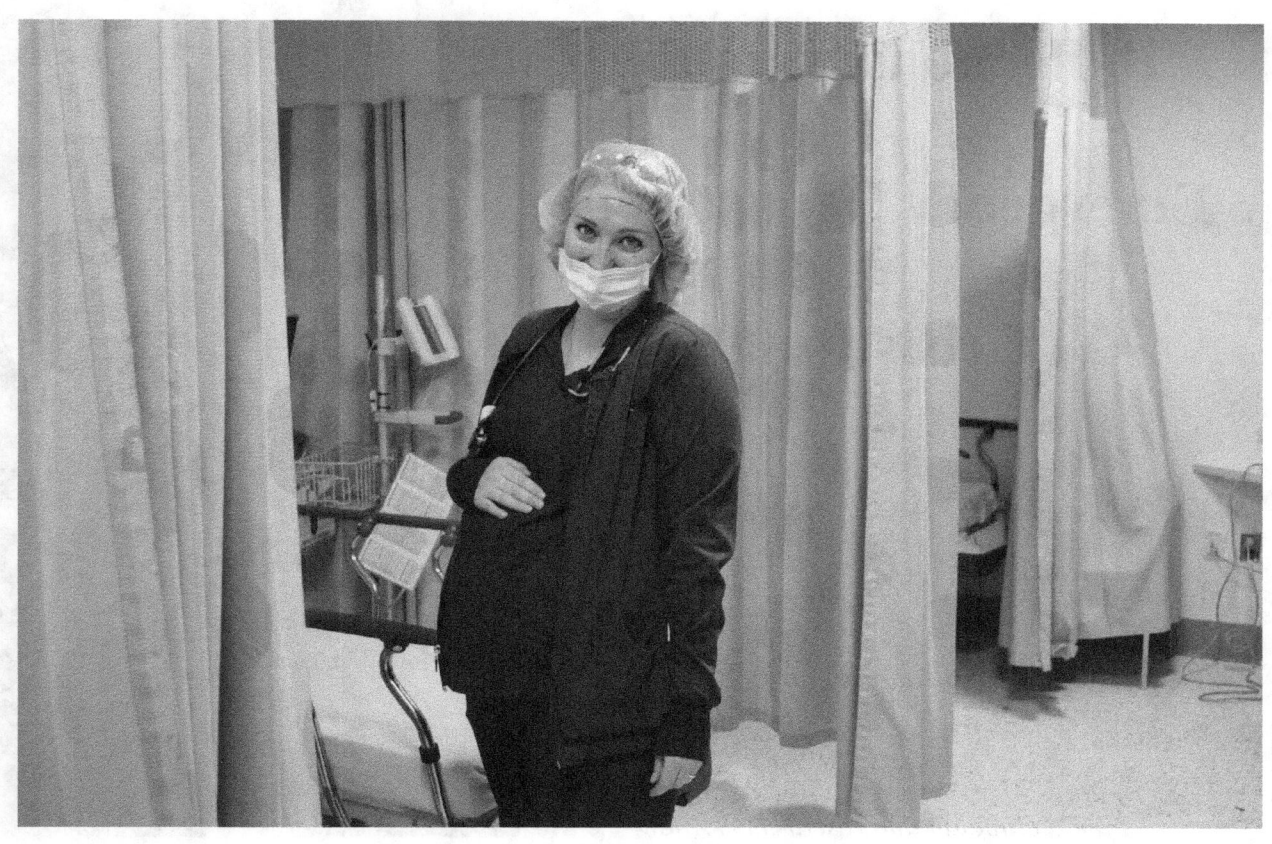

"We are so moved by the outpouring of support from New York City. The applause from balconies, the pizza deliveries and the beautiful crayon art we receive are things we carry with us for a little light on a dark day—and a little strength when we may not feel like superheroes."

- **Lauren Silveira, Registered Nurse, Emergency Department, NYC**

Reflections from the Emergency Department Crisis Unit

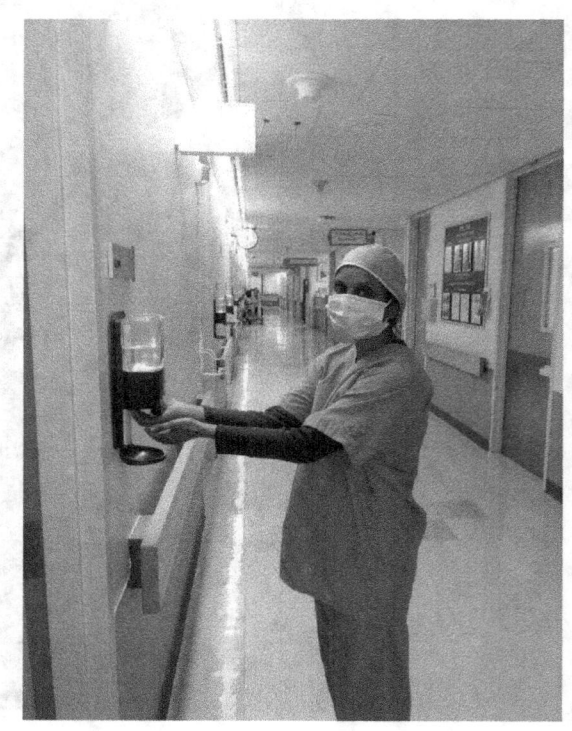

-Dr. Jyothirmayi, PA-C, Emergency Department, Crisis Unit, Dept. of Psychiatry at University Hospital, Newark, NJ

I am a clinician and researcher. A few months ago, I was asked to float at the Crisis Unit in the Emergency Department (ED). Little did I know that I would be on the frontlines taking care of COVID-19 patients during this historic pandemic, at one of the most severely impacted hospitals in New Jersey. For the past three and a half months, my routine is to wake up early with a prayer to God to give me the strength to take care of the needs of my patients and bring me back safely to my family. As I drive through the less crowded streets, my heart is filled with gratitude to people in all walks of life. As I enter the hospital premises and merge with the sea of blue scrubs, I am grateful to the personnel at the hospital entrances checking our temperatures, to the security staff who ensure our safety, and to the staff at the command center who provide us with the *necessary Personal Protective Equipment (PPE) and water to keep us hydrated. I'm thankful to the cafeteria staff who serve us food, to the housekeeping staff who keep up hospital maintenance, to the administrative staff who communicate daily policies and regulations. I am so appreciative for the free food donated by many agencies and the personnel who were kind enough to oversee its distribution. After long, tiring days, as I head home I take a deep breath and give thanks to the amazing doctors, colleagues, nurses, residents, nursing assistants, and the countless other essential personnel who work tirelessly to provide the best possible care to our patients.*

While my family was scared for my safety, I reminded them that I am thankful I have a job where I save lives and that I am honored to be in the company of those who are sacrificing their time and safety to help others. However, when my family sleeps, I realize how exhausted I am from washing my hands every few minutes and eating and sleeping at odd hours. As the days pass, I pray for our patients at every opportunity and try to help as much as I possibly can. During these trying times, I feel emotional whenever people cheer for healthcare and other essential workers. When the Blue Angels and the Thunderbirds soared high in the sky in recognition of our services, I had goosebumps and tears rolling down my cheeks! When the going got tough at the hospital, we were all so appreciative for the timely assistance provided by the Medical Task Force of the U.S. Army Reserve from the 332nd Medical Brigade based at Nashville, Tennessee. I personally had the opportunity to work in the ED Crisis Unit with one of the mental health care clinicians from the U.S. Army. Despite working together for a short period of time, we bonded instantly and I am glad to have made a life-long friend in Tennessee.

While working long hours at the ED Crisis Unit, I felt very honored to provide medical and mental health care to our patients. At times, the ED was filled with people's voices and the bustling of footsteps. Other times, it would be eerily silent with only the sounds of the monitors, which gave us signs of hope and life. At the hospital, our daily routines have evolved from handshakes and hugs to being covered from head to toe in PPE and greeting each other with eye smiles and air hugs while maintaining social distance. Our faith and hope were intermittently shaken by the loss of a patient, a colleague, or a staff member. In those times, we regained strength through prayers and camaraderie. We cheered with music whenever a COVID patient was discharged.

During the past few months, a rollercoaster of emotions was felt by everyone. There were

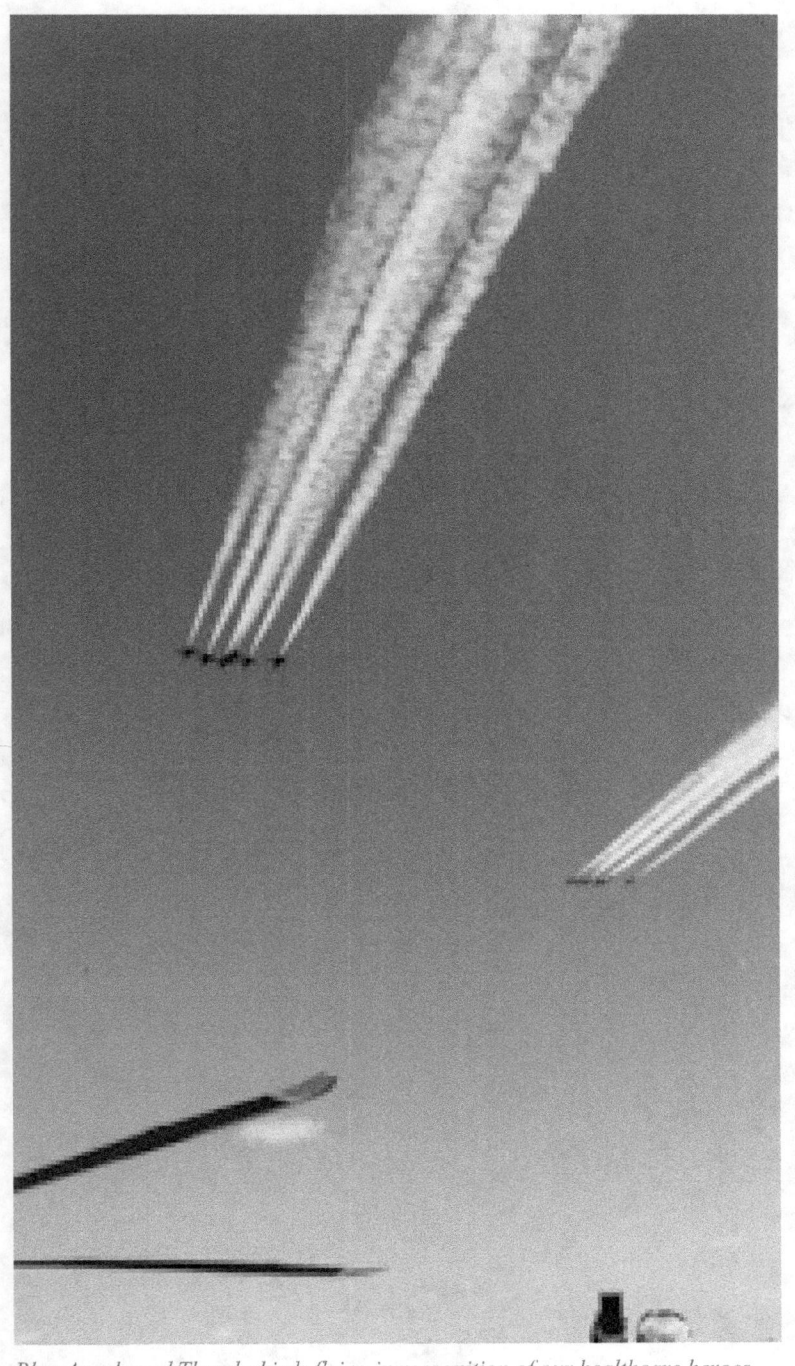

Blue Angels and Thunderbirds flying in recognition of our healthcare heroes

moments of despair where we would hide our tears, and rays of hope that guided us. As a parent, I pray and hope for safe social gathering and time to rejoice with families and friends. As a scientific researcher, I hope to see a vaccine for COVID-19 in the near future. At the end of the day, I am proud and honored to be a healthcare professional, happy for the new friendships made, ever thankful for my family and friends, especially to my dearest daughter, for their kind support, and to Dr. Krutika Parasar Raulkar for giving me this opportunity to mark this unforgettable milestone in my life's journey in the art of science and medicine.

International Perspective: Cape Town, South Africa

—Dr. Yatish Garach, Gastroenterologist

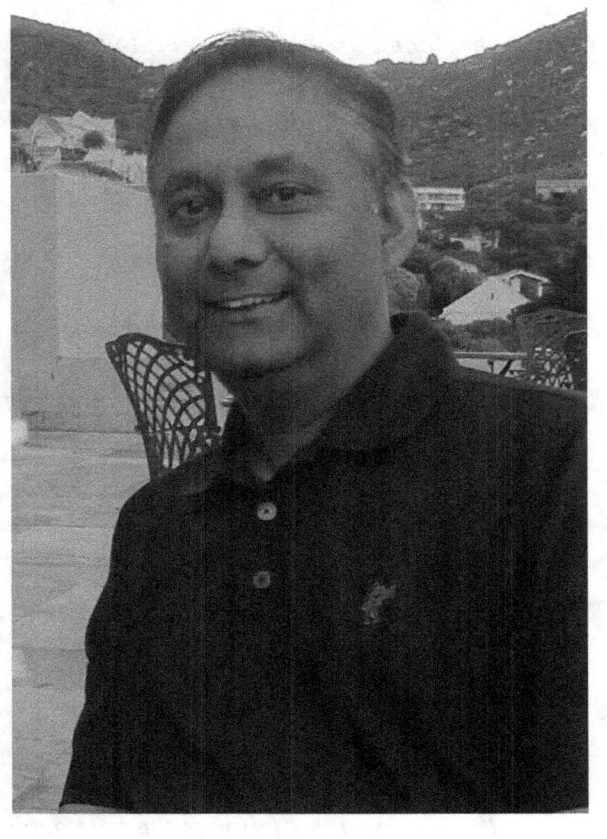

How has the COVID-19 pandemic impacted you personally and professionally? *It has been very stressful and anxiety provoking. I can easily say this pandemic has been the most difficult time of my life. I am a gastroenterologist and my usual work has dried up. Because I have ICU experience, I have been trying to help there as much as possible. There has been a 90% drop in non-COVID patients. The COVID patients are a different kettle of fish. There is a lot to learn. Most of the patients I have seen had mild to moderate disease. But I have had a few patients with severe disease requiring ventilation. Just a handful of them have been able to survive off the ventilator. The mild patients do well upon discharge.*

Did your hospital ever run out of ventilators? *There were some hair-raising days when we found that all the ventilators were being used but somehow the hospital management was able to secure more from other hospitals promptly.*

How do you feel your hospital handled the pandemic? *I think the hospital did a pretty good job providing us with PPE and our hospital in Cape Town has been great. In early March, they immediately stopped all visitation to the hospital. Early on, we decided that any admission coming in for non-COVID procedures would receive screening COVID swabs.*

Why do you think there was a decrease in non-COVID cases? *I don't know the answer to that. We did discourage bookings. We told a lot of patients who had chronic issues that we will see them down the line. I think patients themselves were very scared to come to the hospital.*

What kind of repercussions do you think these patients will face by postponing care? *There will definitely be repercussions, especially for patients with chronic conditions and malignancies. I have had a few IBD patients requiring biologics who elected to postpone therapy, which I felt was the best decision at this time.*

What are your opinions on South Africa's handling of the pandemic? *The initial lockdown that the governing party introduced was quite timely. South Africa is a complicated country. You have people living in a first world environment, and on the other hand people living in worse than third world conditions. This latter population does not have enough medical care due to the long-standing oppression in the country. I feel the current government could have done more to improve their access to healthcare in recent years. This population has been disproportionately affected by the pandemic and is now suffering from cases increasing at an alarming rate.*

Any other thoughts? *I have been practicing now for 30 years and I have never experienced something like this. These are trying and difficult times. This pandemic has laid bare the inequalities of the world and that mankind is not equipped to handle this type of emergency. One of the lessons to be learned is that modern living is not conducive to a healthy lifestyle in terms of diet and exercise.*

I was diagnosed with COVID last week and I passed it on to my wife this week. Early in my career, I got tuberculosis. Being a doctor you are at risk for severe disease.

CHAPTER 7:

RISK FACTORS FOR COVID-19

"The blood that covered so many of them did not come from wounds, at least not from steel or explosives that had torn away limbs. Most of the blood had come from nosebleeds. A few sailors had coughed the blood up. Others had bled from their ears. Some coughed so hard that autopsies would later show they had torn apart abdominal muscles and rib cartilage. And many of the men writhed in agony and delirium; nearly all those able to communicate complained of headache, as if someone were hammering a wedge into their skulls just behind the eyes, and body aches so intense they felt like bones breaking, A few were vomiting, Finally the skin of some sailors had turned unusual colors; some showed just a tinge of blue around their lips or fingertips, but a few looked so dark one could not tell easily if they were Caucasian or Negro. They looked almost black."

-John M. Barry *in The Great Influenza*

Risk factors for COVID-19 include age, living in a nursing home or long care facility, obesity, HTN, diabetes, cancer, chronic lung disease, asthma, and a history of smoking[79,83]. Ninety-five percent of patients who developed COVID-19 had at least one of these comorbidities, and 88% had two[123]. Older age appears to be one of the most significant risk factors[78]. An analysis of Chinese data shows that chance of death is more than 13% for patients 80 and older, 0.15% for patients in their 30s, and close to 0 for patients under age 20[78]. A CDC study reports similar statistics[78]. This may be partly due to a decreased ability to fight the virus in the elderly. Conversely, another lethal aspect of COVID-19 infection is mounting *too much* of a response, which may explain the morbidity in middle-aged patients who are not typically affected as severely by other viral infections[78].

Research suggests that obesity is also a prominent risk factor, particularly for younger people[76]. A *New England Journal of Medicine* study of 363 COVID-19 patients consecutively admitted to two NYC hospitals revealed that the median age of patients was 62.2, 60.6% were male, and 35.8% were obese[77]. The most common symptoms were cough (79.4%), fever (77.1%), dyspnea (56.5%), myalgia (23.8%), diarrhea (23.7%), and nausea and vomiting (19.1%). Ninety percent of patients had lymphopenia, 27% had thrombocytopenia (low platelet count), and many had elevated liver function and inflammatory markers. Between March 3rd and April 10th, 33.1% of these patients required intubation and by April 17th, only 33.1% of these patients were extubated[77]. 10.2% of patients died and 66.2% were discharged from the hospitals[77].

A multicenter study of 105 patients by the American Cancer Society suggests that patients with cancer are three times more likely to die of COVID-19[81,82]. Severe outcomes were most frequent for patients with metastatic cancer or cancer of the blood or lungs.

Patients treated with surgery were at higher risks of adverse events, but this was not the case for patients who received only radiotherapy[82].

Men are dying at higher rates than women, and are more likely to require hospitalization and mechanical intubation[77]. In Italy and Ireland, men account for 70% of COVID-19 infections[78]. Possible explanations are sex difference in immune response (men also have worse outcomes from influenza), and higher rates of alcohol use and smoking that can weaken the immune system.

Minorities and the economically disadvantaged are also disproportionally affected, possibly because these populations have more comorbidities, live in more crowded conditions and often with extended family, and have less access to healthcare. African Americans make up 13% of the population but 27% of patient fatalities across the nation[59]. In California, Latinos comprise 39% of the state population but represent 53% of the states' cases. On May 18th, it was confirmed that the Navajo Nation surpassed NY in per capita rate, despite their extremely strict stay at home orders requiring documentation on company letterhead for those who leave their homes[59]. Doctors Without Borders have been dispatched to New Mexico to assist the Navajo Nation[60].

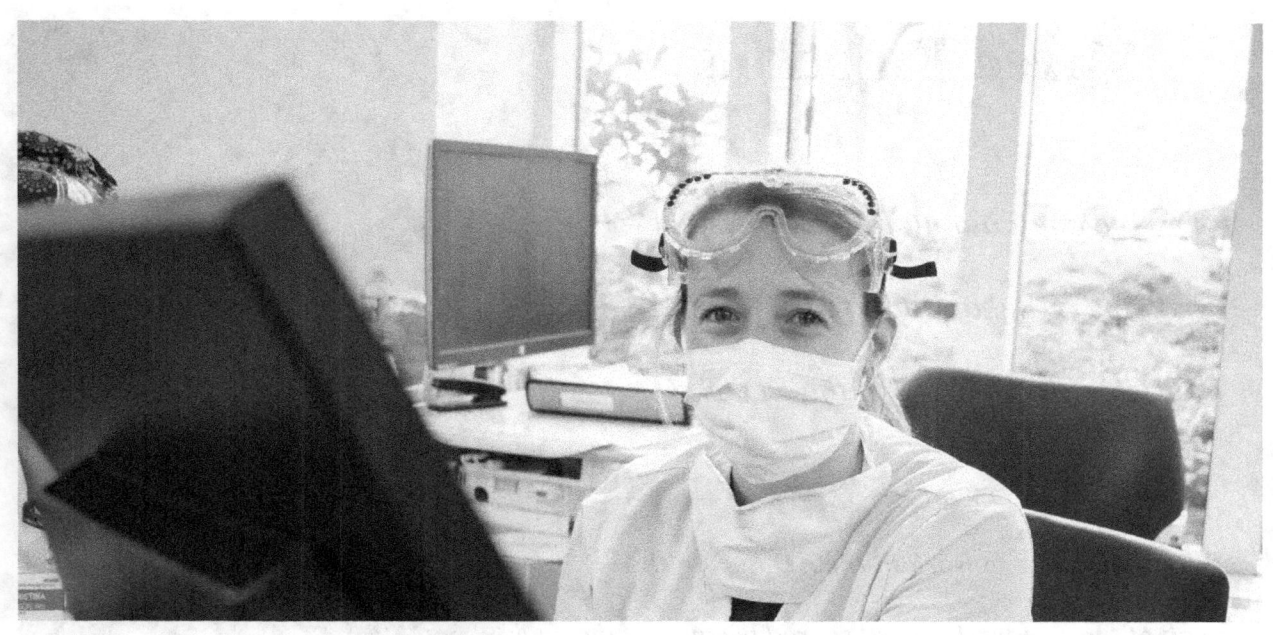

"I'm proud to be part of this amazing team of human beings during this pandemic. We are in this together, we will fight together. Surviving Hurricane Sandy on the frontlines of the ED taught me the importance of camaraderie and teamwork in times of tragedy and hardship. We got this."

-Michelle Penfold, Registered Nurse, Emergency Department, NYC

Mixed Emotions

- Dr. Eugene Palatulan, MD, Physical Medicine & Rehabilitation Resident Physician Redeployed to the ED, NYC

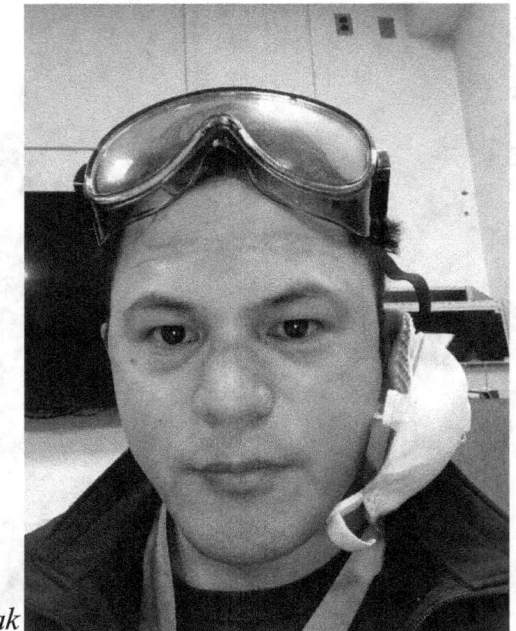

What was it like to work in the ED during the peak of the pandemic? *I felt scared because at the peak by the hundreds in a few hours. COVID patients were in the hallways. You knew they were COVID positive before they tested because they had the symptoms. You could get the x-ray right away and that was diagnostic. I knew I was being exposed to the virus and that was scary. It was also exciting because I got to help and make a difference at the epicenter of the pandemic. It was also sad because I had to stay away from my family for a month, quarantining in hospital-provided housing.*

What was it like to self-quarantine from your wife and daughters? *It was emotionally draining because my wife was still working full time as an OT [occupational therapist] through telemedicine, she also had to take care of the two kids at home, and she is pregnant. I wasn't able to relieve her at the end of the day and she was exhausted. She was definitely the hero of all this. I felt terrible being away from them. I was doing what I was supposed to do because my number was called up and I wasn't going to run away from the responsibility.*

Are there any patient experiences that most affected you? *Definitely. The ones that affected me the most were the young patients without comorbidities.*

What would you like people to know about COVID-19? *This is serious even though forces in society say it's not. It can hurt healthy people too. I wouldn't be too cavalier about not wearing a mask and maintaining hygiene.*

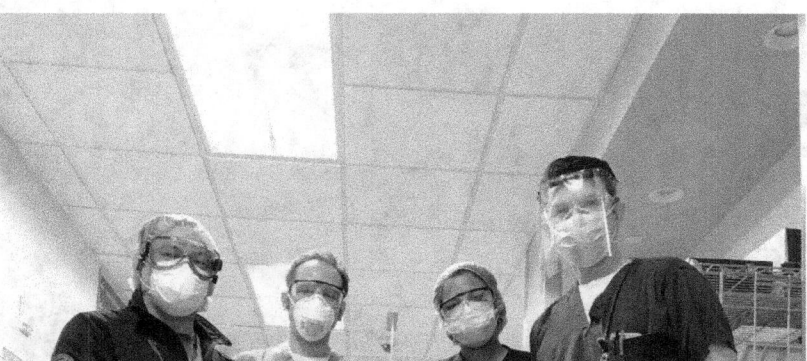

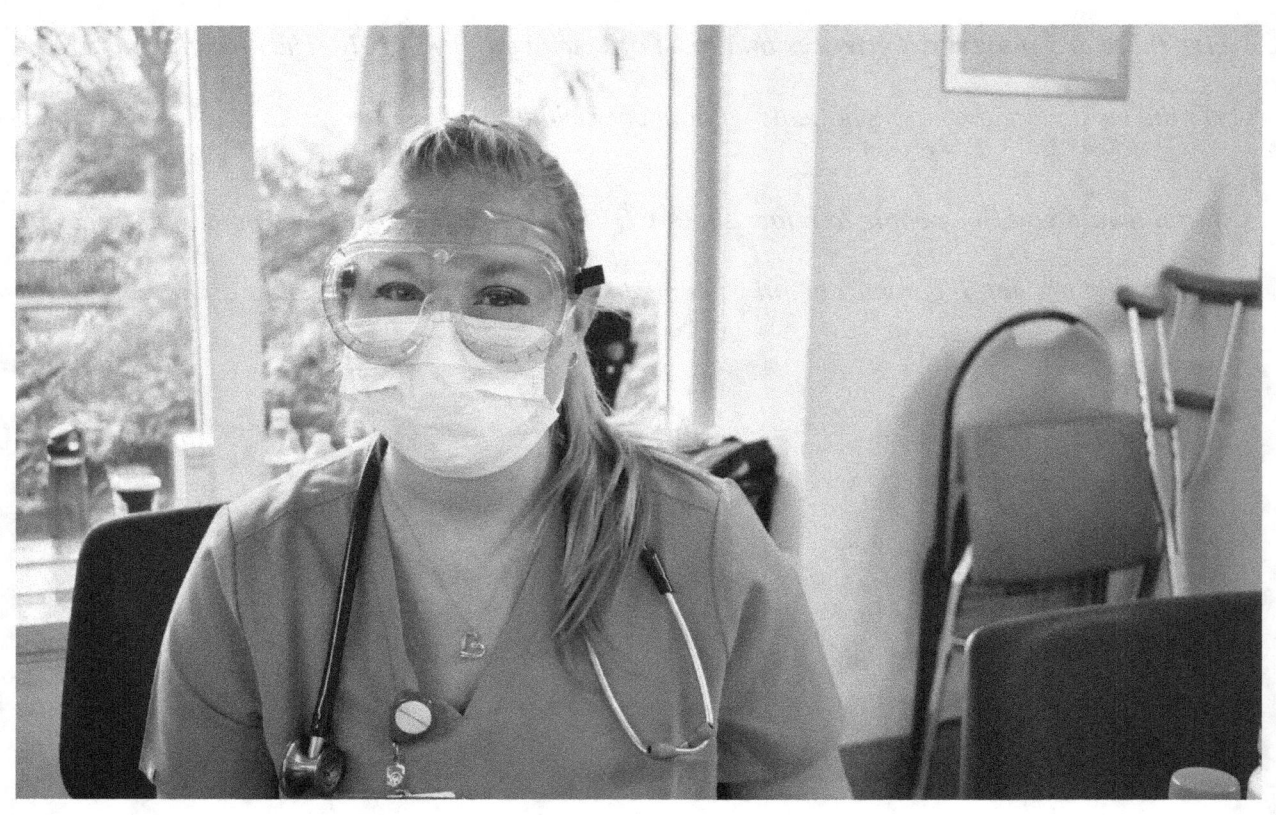

"Today is my first day back after recovering from COVID myself. All I could think about while I was home was about how proud I am of my colleagues holding down the frontline and how I could not wait to get back and fight alongside them all. They're all an inspiration to me. We are in this together. And I truly believe that together we will help bring the world out of the darkness and into the light." **-Kelly Brissenden, Emergency Medicine Physician's Assistant, NYC**

International Perspective: Singapore

—Kalpa Mahender

When the virus began crossing china's borders in January, Singapore appeared fated for a large-scale outbreak. The tiny city-state was the third country to report cases of Covid-19 and by mid-February, recorded over 80 infections, the highest outside the Chinese mainland.

The timing of the emergence of coronavirus could not have been any worse for Singapore, an international travel hub that gets its share of millions of Chinese tourists out and about during the Lunar New Year holidays, the world's largest annual human migration.

There were lessons learned the hard way from the 2003 SARS outbreak which had a significant impact on lives and livelihoods and from which the country took years to recover. Singapore has since been preparing both in terms of building infrastructure and designing legislation in case of a potential outbreak.

By February 1st, Singapore proactively implemented travel restrictions on passengers coming from mainland China. The precautions came at a significant economic cost. The return of Singaporeans, residents, and students from other parts of the world led to a spike which then spread widely in the community despite the containment measures. As Singapore and the world continued to grapple with Covid-19 in the coming weeks, the unforeseen challenge that lay ahead was the unfortunate spread of infection in the many dormitories that host over 600,000 foreign workers mainly in the construction industry.

Post-SARS, Singapore had developed facilities that could detect three times more cases than the global average due to its strong surveillance and fastidious contact tracing. Given the spread in dormitories, testing was significantly increased and that resulted in positives cases crossing 50,000 by the middle of July. There have been 27 deaths to date, which remains relatively low compared to rest of the world. I believe this is due to the advanced healthcare facilities that the country has established over the years.

Quarantine, isolation, and social distancing protocols were strictly enforced in our island of 5.7 million people. Between early April and mid-June, we entered our 1st phase of what was called a circuit breaker that prevented any social contact outside the household, and closure of all non-essential services and schools. Students began home-based learning as parents juggled between zoom conferences. Essential services remained open, and individuals were allowed to exercise around the neighborhood. Masks were made mandatory with an exception if one is doing strenuous exercise such as running or cycling.

Those breaching quarantine and social distancing rules, or providing false information about their travel history, were given strict punishments including jail term, penalties, or their work permits withdrawn and deported back to the country of origin.

Prime minister Lee Hsien Loong's frequent address to the public reinforced the trust he has established with the citizens and residents alike. His open and transparent messages on the need to be vigilant and not to panic was reciprocated by all. There was no politicizing of the situation. People were cooperative with the safe distancing measures during the strict implementation of the circuit breaker and after the restrictions were removed in mid-June.

The Singapore Government WhatsApp messaging group became the one-stop source for accurate information and dispelling any rumors.

The contact tracing mobile apps, which most people willingly installed, helped leave a digital signature and made contact tracing a lot easier and quicker than elsewhere. Whilst the contact tracing was largely successful, many cases were still being missed, resulting in community spread.

It's been over a month since the circuit breaker restrictions have been lifted. People are allowed to attend social gatherings of not more than five guests at home. Bars and restaurants can now host groups of five at a table and retail businesses have resumed operations with clear social distancing guidance. Schools reopened once again for a couple of weeks before the term ended, which was a welcome relief for students who were bereft of any social interaction beyond the zoom classroom sessions.

The economic toll has been significant and the recovery may take years, but the government has done a commendable job in supporting small businesses and livelihoods by releasing funds from its reserves.

We are a family of four and permanent residents of Singapore. We find ourselves extremely fortunate to be here in Singapore rather than any other place in the world at this moment. We live within a largely responsible community that recognizes the need to follow social distancing and remain vigilant to the devastating effects of a pandemic that has impacted millions across the world. Perhaps there is a lot the world can learn from the resilience of the Singapore people and its leadership as it continues to maneuver through the ups and downs of the new, uncertain world in which we are living.

CHAPTER 8: TESTING FOR COVID-19

"Woo! That's wicked"

"That's weird"

"I feel like your touching my brain"

"I'm sorry for being such a baby"

Some patients laughed at the "uncomfortable sensation," while most reflexively teared, including myself.

During the week of May 11th, my colleagues and I performed the nasopharyngeal swab on all the patients and employees in an acute care rehabilitation hospital. When I transitioned to the VA, I participated in testing of patients on a biweekly basis.

There has been much attention in the media to obtain more tests to get a better sense of who is getting COVID-19, and so those infected can quarantine themselves. The high testing rate in America, and in particular NYC, is likely one factor that explains why we have so many cases as compared to other countries. Governors have reiterated the need for testing capacity before they can safely open their states. As the pandemic progressed, testing became much more available, enabling contact tracing and better containment of spread.

What kind of tests are available?

There are two tests typically administered. One is a nasopharyngeal (NP) swab, similar to a flu swab, that directly detects the COVID-19 antigen. This can tell you if you are actively infected with COVID-19. It is performed by inserting the swab deep into the nasopharyngeal space, where the concentration of the virus in highest.

The second is an antibody test that tells you whether you have mounted an immune response to the virus. When your body is exposed to a virus, it produces immediate IgM antibodies to bind and deactivate the viral antigen. After 14 days, it produces IgG antibodies that confer memory to the viral antigens, so you can quickly defeat them next time your body sees them. This confers long-lasting immunity. The antibody test is a serum test that can detect the level of IgG in your blood so it will only be positive 14 days after you are exposed, and the further from exposure that you are tested, the more likely you will have a positive response. As SARS-CoV-2 is a novel coronavirus, we do not know whether these antibodies disappear over time; thus, we do not know if immunity is long-lasting for this virus. Current data suggests that immunity lasts for 2-3 months. In comparison, for the closely related SARS-CoV-1, immunity appeared to last for 3 years. For many strains of the flu, immunity only lasts for 1 year[26], which is why a yearly vaccine is recommended. Furthermore, some evidence suggests that children and asymptomatic adults may not mount any antibody response[27] and thus may test negative while still being able to spread the virus.

The antigen test is most useful when you have symptoms or if you have been in contact with someone exposed. The antibody test is more helpful if you have had symptoms or been exposed to someone in the past. In May, NY tested grocery store shoppers and found that

20% were positive for COVID-19. It is estimated that 60% of the population must be exposed to achieve herd immunity.

What is herd immunity?

Herd immunity describes when a large chunk of the population has immunity to a pathogen and thus people who cannot be immunized (in the case of COVID, our elderly and patients with comorbidities) can be protected by others who are immunized. This concept is also used in vaccination. The majority of the population is vaccinated and herd immunity is achieved; those who cannot be vaccinated for medical reasons can still be safe because the disease cannot easily spread to them.

In late May, results from studies around the world reveal that immunity rates remain in the single digits in many countries. This suggests that herd immunity is still a long way off[96]. In the United States, highest positivity rates have been found in Chelsea, Massachusetts (32%), NYC (25%)[117]. Many areas have positivity rates less than 3%.

How accurate are COVID-19 tests[24]?

Two terms are frequently used to describe a test's accuracy- sensitivity and specificity. Sensitivity describes the ability of a test to *rule out* a condition whereas specificity describes its ability to *rule in* a condition. Although COVID-19 NP swabs tend to be specific, several factors influence their sensitivity, including a person's biology, the reagent used to test, and performance of the test with proper technique (i.e. holding the swab deep in the nasopharynx of *each* nostril for a total of 10 seconds at a time). This means that if you get a positive result it is likely true; if you get a negative result there is a good chance it is false. To increase sensitivity, NP swabs should be performed as close to symptom onset as possible[25].

Antibody tests are thought to be specific in 82-100% of cases and sensitive in 91-100% of cases[117]. Despite these relatively high numbers, I have spoken to many healthcare providers with extensive, daily exposure to COVID-19 infected patients, who have not mounted antibodies. I received the antibody test from NYP on 6/16/20. My blood was drawn at 1:02 pm, and by 4:05pm I had my result: negative. Is it PPE that is protecting us from COVID-19 despite our significant exposure? After investigating literature and discussing with colleagues, I believe we may not be mounting antibodies because we are able to successfully defeat the virus with a T cell response and thus do not form enough antibodies to be detected by serum testing. Although the body often mounts both a T cell and B cell (antibody) response against invaders, often one of these responses is more effective against a particular pathogen. In the case of both coronaviruses and influenza viruses, the T cell response is thought to be the most important. Unfortunately, this response is not as easy to measure. But this may mean that the antibody tests we are relying on to assess levels of immunity is not an accurate indicator of exposure, as many of us may have been exposed to the virus and easily defeated it with a cellular immune response. Despite this, it is still unclear whether we will achieve herd immunity easily, given that we do not know how long immunity to COVID-19 lasts. Some scientists predict that COVID-19 could become an endemic disease- so we may have a COVID-19 season in addition to a flu season every year[122].

When should I be tested?

If you have symptoms of COVID-19, you should stay home and self-quarantine to avoid spreading the disease to others. If you would like, you can obtain a self-test kit to test yourself while at home. If your healthcare provider recommends that you be tested, they may ask you to come in for a swab. Many hospitals are testing all their admitted patients. All three hospitals where I worked during the pandemic followed this procedure. As per our policy in the free-standing rehabilitation center, I retested every admission to our unit, even if they had tested negative at their discharging hospital. This helped to ensure appropriate isolation of COVID-19 patients to minimize spread to vulnerable hospital patients.

Why shouldn't everyone be tested?

Initially swabs were limited. Now we have more, but doing mass testing would overwhelm the labs that process the swabs. Thus, tests are still being provided on a controlled basis only after determined necessary by a healthcare provider. This may change in the future, as the spread of the virus slows. The Trump Administration has said they will work with retailers like Walmart and Target to offer drive-through tests at their locations[46].

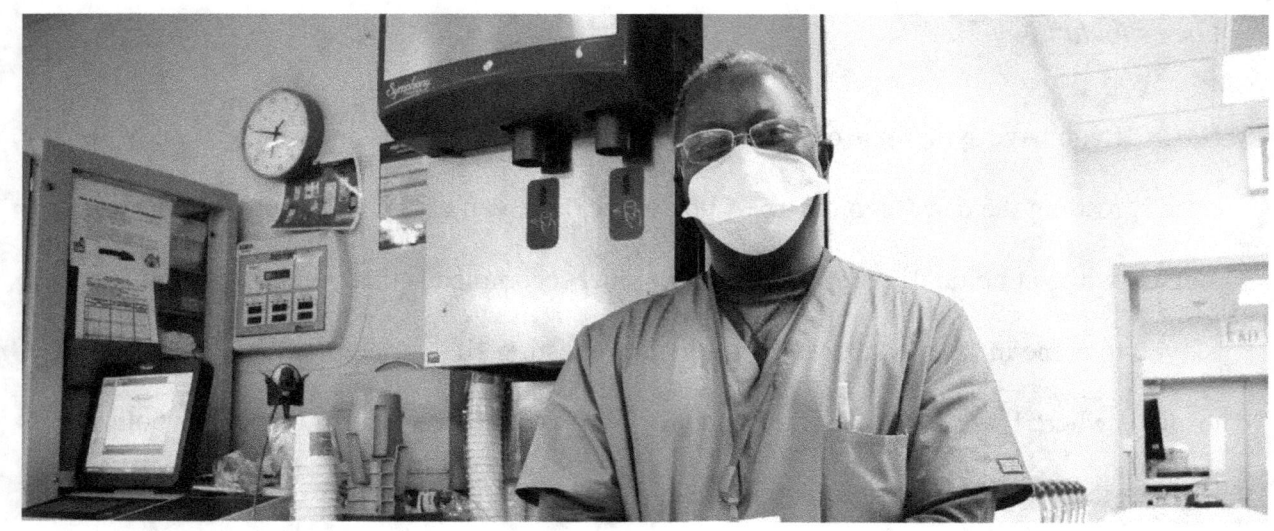

"Take care of yourself."

-Kasper, Mental Health Provider, NYC

Reflections from a Speech Language Pathologist (SLP), NYC

-Talia Schwartz, MS-CCC-SLP, NYC

Modified from original version published on DysphagiaCafé.com on April 22, 2020

When our hospital admitted the first NY case of COVID-19 in the beginning of March, we felt uneasy—but nothing around us really changed, and we all went about our business as usual. Then in what felt like the blink of an eye, the COVID-19 admissions started rolling in, the PPE guidelines started changing, and the streets of NYC started shutting down. We braced ourselves.

Our first patient was extubated and our SLP service was consulted for a dysphagia evaluation. We paused. There's got to be data from China or Italy on what to do, right? After reaching out to contacts abroad- we realized there really wasn't information to guide us. Right around that time, CDC guidelines came out to avoid endoscopic procedures.

A month later, we are smack in the center of COVID-land and our SLP service is responding to consults left and right. I know that some are questioning if our service is essential in treatment of these patients. I will just say that at our hospital, SLP, PT, and OT are all hands-on deck.

So how are we managing? What types of COVID-19 patients are we seeing and how are they faring? What are we doing without objective assessment? I wanted to share some honest reflections to these questions.

How are we managing?

- PPE: *For all COVID-19 patient contact: every SLP is wearing an N95 respirator, with a surgical mask on top (for conservation of the N95), protective glasses, a face shield, gown, and gloves.*
- Staffing: *Our hospital provides 7-day/week SLP coverage: We have staggered our work shifts from 5 short days to 4 long days in efforts to prevent office overcrowding, limit the number of days we need to commute on public transportation, allow more time to respond to lengthy consults, and have an additional day off for mental health.*
- Consults: *In our effort to reduce exposure and preserve PPE, we are carefully triaging each case and talking to the medical team first: is the patient ready for our evaluation? Can we make a reasonable recommendation (perhaps after chart review, discussion with the nurse, contact with the patient's family or nursing home, etc.) without entering the room?*

What types of COVID19 patients are we seeing?

Post-Extubation

- *We recently had what felt like the first wave of consults of patient post-extubation, and now it feels like a steady stream. Currently, our hospital system has over 750 patients in the ICUs on ventilators. What are the trends with these post-extubation cases? There aren't any! Some have an extensive past medical history, others have none. The length of intubation varies from 3 days to 3 weeks. We have evaluated patients aged 32 to 82. Some patients have been proned, others haven't.*
- *Initially one thing remained the same- we got consulted right after the tube came out. Our service is not performing videographic dysphagia studies, so we educated our physicians on post-extubation dysphagia considerations, and have developed guidelines that we wait at least 24 hours before assessment given the increased risk for laryngeal sensory deficits. We have also asked that NGTs [nasogastric tubes] remain or be placed upon extubation if it is anticipated that the patient will need immediate access to critical medications or is elderly with many comorbidities.*

- *What do these patients look like? Some have been aphonic, full of secretions, and seem peri-reintubation. Others patients are borderline- perhaps slightly dysphonic and weak but look like they have potential for some oral intake. We have used our bedside clinical judgement here. Yes, we acknowledge this is subjective and we discuss the limitations with our physicians. We have initiated many patients on modified diets and thickened liquids. But if we can't definitively rule out aspiration of thickened liquids, isn't it safer to aspirate water? We recognize this, but sometimes have felt a consistent choking response to thin liquids just isn't ok. We have been somewhat conservative with our diet texture recommendations and consider the patient's comorbidities, hospital course, general presentation, etc.*
- *How are these patients faring? Looking back so far: some of those peri-reintubation patients were indeed re-intubated, some passed away. Some of those patients fully recovered, we advanced their diet, and they returned home. Others have been discharged to nursing facilities on dysphagia diets.*
- *We now have access to MBS [Modified Barium Swallow] on a case by case basis and will reserve this for patients with a history that really suggests high risk for silent aspiration- like stroke, head and neck cancer, prior trach, or those with suspected vocal fold trauma post-extubation that doesn't resolve.*

Hypoxia

- *Our institution is treating hypoxia due to COVID19 with non-rebreather masks (NRB), as opposed to high flow nasal cannula or BiPAP- in efforts to create a seal during oxygen delivery and reduce aerosol generation.*
- *But what about eating and drinking? Perhaps our most challenging battle has been educating medical teams about the implications of desaturating and increased work of breathing with NRB removal to eat and drink- by altering respiratory/swallow coordination and increasing aspiration risk.*
- *Our service has deferred consults received when a patient is requiring an NRB and recommending NPO [nothing by mouth]- we will assess the patient when stable and weaned to nasal cannula. We keep in mind that some of these physicians are specialists now being asked to manage COVID patients and do our best to educate. In a preliminary review of 27 consults that were deferred as the patient required an NRB at the time: 22 out of the 27 then expired. This would seem to support*

appropriateness of deferrals. But what about those patients we are not consulted on that eat/drink in this fashion and seem to do A-ok?

Altered Mental Status/Dementia

- *Excluding ICU delirium- we have seen a significant amount of patients coming in with altered mental status in the setting of metabolic disarray from poor oral intake, or with lethargy in the setting of infection. We are frequently seeing this in the dementia population, and elderly patients with significant comorbidities.*
- *These cases are tough (and sad). From a safety perspective, it has seemed quite obvious that this patient whose mental status is significantly altered is at high risk for aspiration. NPO! But we realized that COVID19 is quickly tipping many of these patients over the edge.*
- *We recently talked with our palliative care team about early clarification of goals of care in regards to eating/drinking when families discuss DNR/DNI. We are asking about the patient's prognosis, and if it is poor, we are suggesting teams liberalize comfort feeds to align with the patient's goals.*

Other Diagnoses

- *Stroke: more and more literature is coming out about potential neurological consequences of COVID-19. We have continued to see stroke patients, as well as patients with recrudescence of their old stroke symptoms in setting of the infection.*
- *Trachs: We are now performing tracheostomies for patients after prolonged intubations. We are in ongoing discussions with our surgeons and critical care teams to discuss candidates and what post trach care and SLP intervention will look like.*

This is a broad glimpse into SLP/COVID-land at my hospital-it is definitely not exclusive. In some ways- treating COVID-19 patients has been no different than treating other cases. We are using clinical judgement, critical thinking skills, and communicating with medical teams- as we always have done. We are still faced with the same challenges: NPO vs comfort feeds? Aspiration vs dehydration/ hypernatremia risk? Every patient is unique- we make recommendations on a case by case basis.

But in other ways- our practice has drastically changed to accommodate the COVID19 situation. We are relying heavily on our bedside skills given the lack of access to instrumental assessment. We are deferring assessments until we feel the patient presentation is optimized. We stopped ambulatory appointments very early on and have transitioned to televisits for our outpatients.

This has been a challenging experience, and we know it is far from over. Our team has the support of our institution which provides shuttles to work, supplies PPE, provides meals, and is transparent with updates. Our department meets frequently (socially-distanced of course!) to discuss case management, reflect on our data, and support each other.

In sharing some insight, the hope is to open the doors for discussion, ideas, collaboration, etc. And if anyone knows how to talk under an N95 without getting winded, please share!

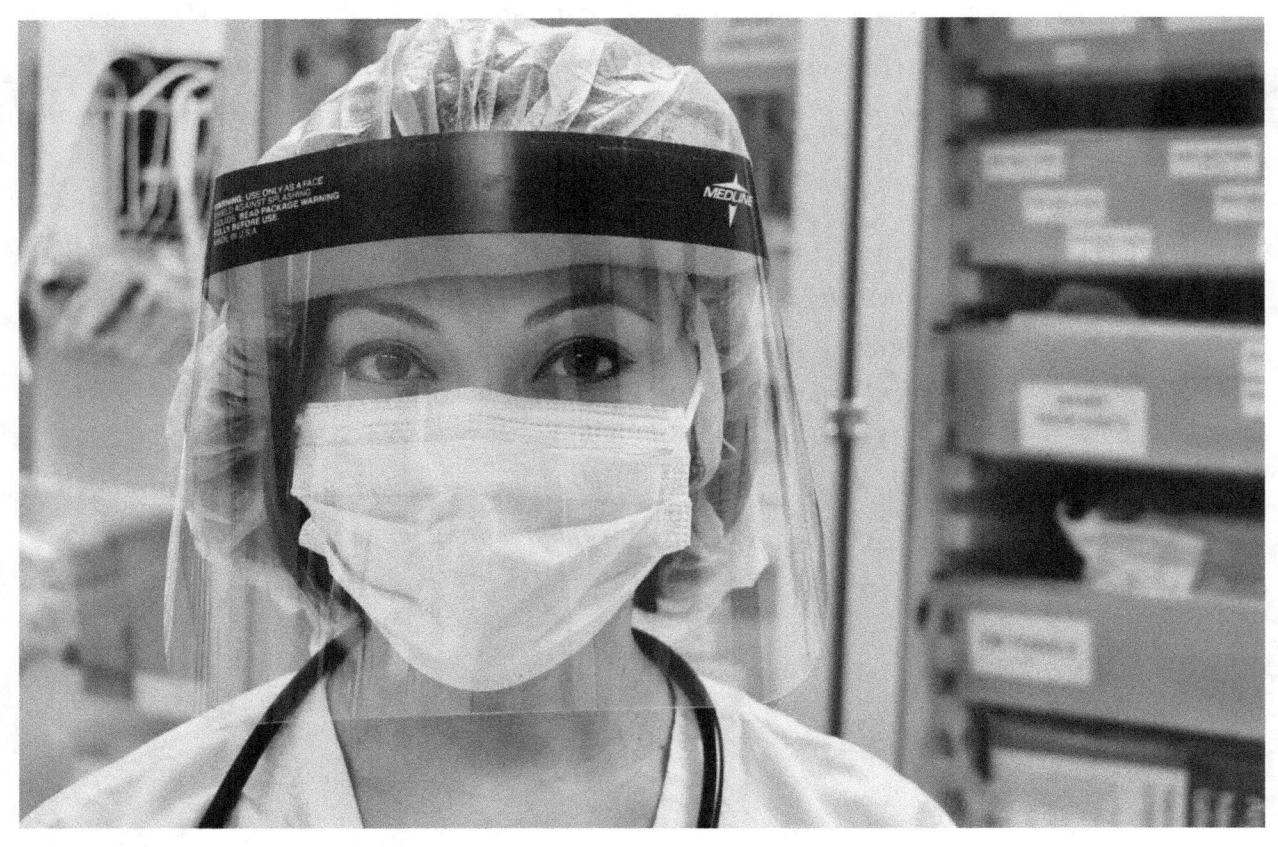

"Through our good days, busy days, and extremely challenging days, I know I don't go through it alone. We go through hurricanes, literally and figuratively, together."

- Sara Choi, Registered Nurse, Emergency Department, NYC

International Perspective—Portugal

Nandini Singla—Indian Ambassador to Portugal

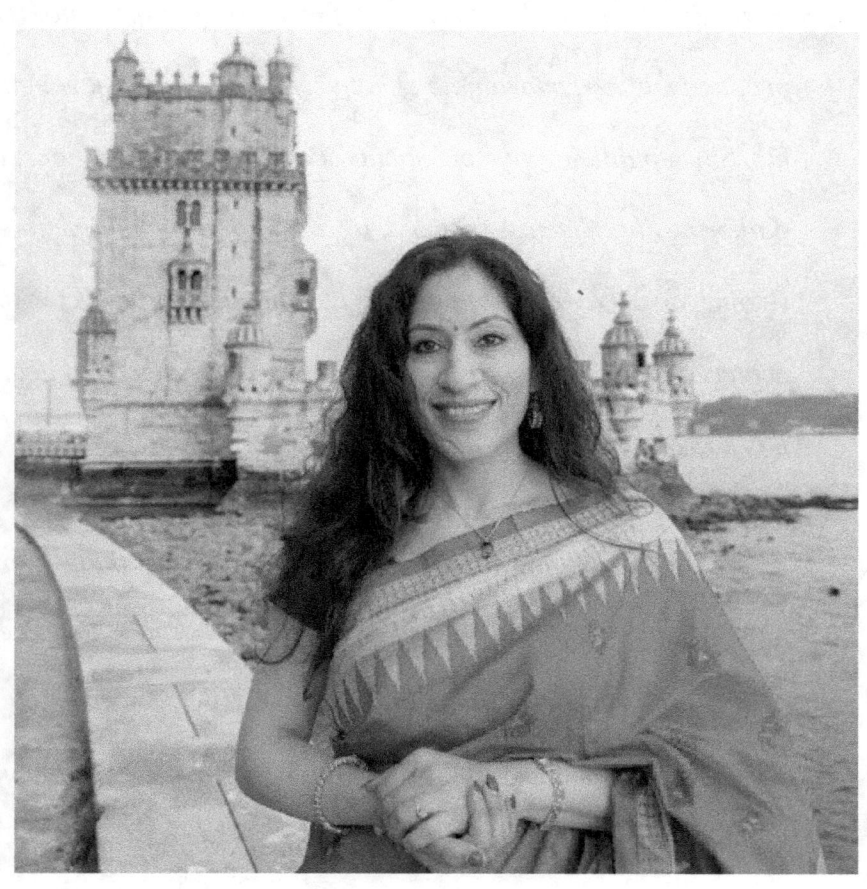

How has the pandemic affected you personally and professionally? The pandemic has changed a lot of things in terms of values, lifestyle, our priorities, and the ways in which we work and live. For me, it has brought quite a few revelations. At the personal level, we have family living across continents. My husband is the Indian Ambassador to Israel and lives in Tel Aviv. My younger son lives with him and goes to school there. I'm in Portugal with my dog, and our older son goes to Swarthmore College, outside of Philadelphia. Early in March, he became very ill in the U.S. with a high fever, a severe sore throat, difficulty swallowing, and swollen lymph nodes in his neck. People were not fully aware of Covid at that time and he was advised to see a cancer specialist. We were worried and I was considering flying out to get him myself. Eventually, we decided to fly him out to Israel since Covid-19 was rapidly spreading across Europe then.

In Portugal, a State of Emergency was declared in March. Our Embassy had to shift to online services for our public work related to visas, passports, and consular services. We cut down staff and asked those taking public transport to work from home. Personally, working from home has been one of my best life experiences. I found that I was able to work productively and coordinate effectively with my team through daily group calls, chats, emails etc. Since public events and social occasions like receptions, dinners and diplomatic gatherings had been suspended, it was an opportune time to go on a fitness and exercise regime, do Yoga, meditate and go for long evening walks with my dog. I feel fitter, more centered and happier! By the grace of God, my near and dear ones are doing fine and no one has had significant health problems.

On the work front, the pandemic has shown that we are capable of creatively adapting to rapidly evolving and uncertain situations to find innovative ways of ensuring that public services are rendered efficiently and humanely. For instance, we set up a new online system during the pandemic called "Sampark" to provide all our consular services digitally. We are now trying to go fully digital to avoid the challenge of people coming physically to the Embassy for consular services.

At a human level, I have seen the pandemic bring out the best in the human spirit. In Portugal, we have about 120,000 people of Indian origin. A lot of them are Indian passport holders who work in Portugal temporarily, in the agricultural sector, construction industry, etc. A lot of them suddenly lost their jobs due to the pandemic and didn't have places to live or even food to eat. Despite the Emergency situation, our Embassy staff managed to deliver food to over 2,000 people, mostly through local Indian diaspora and Indian community organizations. Our Embassy in Lisbon has limited staff and we don't have Consulates or subsidiary offices anywhere in Portugal; therefore, reaching out to volunteers and enlisting their help, was the key to delivering the urgently-needed assistance. I was humbled and amazed by the heroic and humanitarian spirit I saw when people offered to risk their lives and their wellbeing to serve others in distress. For instance, in southern Portugal where we had about 70 infected Indian farm workers, the Portuguese authorities quarantined all those who were working alongside them, in a local school for 14 days. In cases where they were taken straight from their farms to the isolation centers, the Indian workers called the Embassy requesting supply of clothes, footwear, toiletries, Indian food, Indian tea etc. We were able to arrange all these immediately only because of the ready assistance of our Indian friends living in the area who courageously volunteered to help. To me, these bravehearts are truly 'COVID warriors' because some of them actually wore Hazmat suits and went to these quarantined centers and personally distributed food, tea kettles, milk, tea powder, footwear, toiletries, clothes. They also helped interpret communication between the Portuguese authorities and the Punjabi-speaking Indian workers. Last week, as a token of our appreciation and gratitude, I gave 'Covid Warrior' certificates to these volunteers on behalf of the Embassy.

It sounds like you were much busier during the pandemic. How did you manage to care for people while working remotely? Yes, we were much busier and it was a challenge to execute unprecedented support operations remotely. Fellow Indians living in Portugal were getting anxious about their health and safety; those who had lost their jobs were worried about their survival and were growing desperate; many who were stranded in Portugal wanted to go back to their families in India. We realized, right at the outset, that communication was the *key. So, we used the Embassy's website, social media channels, phones and emails to calm and reassure all Indians in Portugal and regularly update them about relevant new regulations and announcements of the Portuguese and Indian governments. For instance, I made a WhatsApp Video message myself in Hindi, outlining protocols to be followed in case of Covid-19 symptoms, hospitals to go to, and reassuring them that all foreigners would be treated on par with Portuguese citizens in terms of healthcare even in the absence of a valid Portuguese visa. As you can imagine, we were inundated by an overwhelming number of queries on our Emergency phone, WhatsApp, Email etc. I am proud to say that we answered each and every query in a personalized way and responded to over 4,000 messages. We managed to send around 100 people back to India through flights arranged by the Indian government.*

In another case, we had a cruise ship docked in Lisbon for more than a couple of months, with 191 Indian seafarers on board. They called the Embassy saying they were very anxious regarding the lack of masks, food, social distancing and Wi-Fi connectivity to speak to their families in India. We got in touch with the cruise company and they provided individual rooms, good food, masks, hand sanitizers, Wi Fi etc. Our seafarers were very happy and even made YouTube videos thanking the Embassy. It was very satisfying for me and my team to see the difference we could make in making our people feel safer and taken care of, in a foreign land at a time of crisis.

Your team did amazing work. Can you speak to the timeline of the lockdown in Portugal? And were there repeat lockdowns in response to more cases of the virus? *The lockdown started in early March. It was fortunate that Portugal was behind the curve in terms of the* *peak of the infection and people had the time to learn from the experiences of other European countries like Italy and Spain. The Portuguese government wisely announced a timely and decisive lockdown and enforced it well; the Portuguese people were also cooperative. With Portugal recording 1/5 the mortality rate of Spain and registering far fewer cases, Portugal has managed things well and succeeded in containing the pandemic so far. Hospital beds are not filling up to capacity and the country has spare healthcare workers and resources to tap into, in the event of a second wave.*

The state of Emergency was lifted on 3rd May by the Portuguese government and restrictions were relaxed. As restaurants reopened and people resumed traveling and mingling, as in other countries, Portugal saw a rise in cases, especially around Lisbon. In response, the government reinstated stricter regulations on 1st July. A 'State of Calamity' was declared in 19 most-affected Parishes whereby not more than 5 people could gather together. A 'State of Contingency' was announced in the Lisbon metropolitan area, barring gatherings of more than 10 people. In the rest of Portugal, not more than 20 people can get together. On 30th July, the 'State of Calamity' in the 19 Parishes was lifted and substituted by a 'State of Contingency'. The government continues to carefully monitor the situation. The Prime Minister has signaled about the low probability of another lockdown to avoid further deleterious effects on the economy and has cautioned about a potential second wave in winter when immunity is likely to be low and conditions more conducive to virus spread. My sense is that people are learning to live with Covid-19; they will continue to wear masks and follow necessary precautions as life returns to normalcy.

That's great they are planning ahead. In what ways has the government provided for the people most severely impacted by the virus? *The government has announced several financial aid packages to mitigate the impact of Covid-19 on the Portuguese people, starting with a 9.2-billion-euro package in March which enabled those who had lost their jobs to continue to receive 2/3 of their wages. A stimulus package has also been announced to create new jobs and boost the economy. Since nearly 17% of Portugal's GDP comes from tourism and hospitality which have taken a big hit during the pandemic, these are likely to be important focus sectors.*

The Portuguese government also automatically extended all expired visas which was a big help to foreign immigrants and stranded tourists. The Government also announced that everyone residing in Portugal would be treated as Portuguese nationals, thereby allowing all foreigners to access the Portuguese public healthcare system.

Anything else you would like to add? *India and Portugal have very good relations and this was strengthened during the pandemic. For instance, the Indian government helped repatriate many stranded Portuguese back to Portugal. Also, at Portugal's request, India lifted the ban on export of 2.5 million tablets of Hydroxychloroquine (HCQ) tablets for Portugal's use. The Prime Ministers of India and Portugal spoke on the phone on May 5th. They exchanged notes and reiterated their support to each other's countries in countering the pandemic. Both countries will be anchoring a virtual youth Hack-a-thon in October with COVID as the theme, to find innovative ways of managing, treating and curing COVID-19. This is a new initiative for both countries.*

CHAPTER 9:

PREVENTION OF COVID-19

"We're seeing that with social distancing interventions, it's reduced transmission rate, reduced the likelihood of transmission to somewhere between 0.6 and 1. So now each infected individual is infecting less than one new person. This means that eventually you're breaking that transmission, you're reducing that epidemic."

- Dr. Natasha Martin, Ph. D[66]

How Can You Prevent Getting COVID-19?

1) Limit exposure. Stay at home if you are able.

2) Social distance. Stay 6 feet away from other people to prevent the spread of the virus through air droplets.

3) If you can't social distance, wear a mask. If you are a healthcare worker, wear a mask at all times. *You should not wear a mask if you have trouble breathing or are unable to remove the mask without assistance.*

4) Wash your hands for 20 seconds before eating, after sneezing, and after using the bathroom.

5) Try not to touch your eyes, mouth, and nose.

6) Disinfect items you bring into your home, including groceries and mail.

Can Drinking Hot Liquids Kill the Disease?

No. Once the virus enters your mouth, it can reach your lungs. It cannot be killed by hot water gargling or consuming hot liquids[57].

When Should I See a Doctor?

If you have unremitting fever, lethargy, or worsening shortness of breath, you should absolutely contact your healthcare provider for a video consult. Even if your symptoms are mild, it does not hurt to seek the advice of your doctor by phone or video chat. They can help you determine whether you should stay at home or whether your symptoms are severe enough that you should go to the clinic or emergency room. The CDC also recommends consulting your doctor if you have been exposed to someone with COVID-19 or if you have travelled to a region with high COVID-19 rates.

For How Long Will We Have to Social Distance?

This will be determined on a state-by-state basis depending on rates of infection and mortality and when cases peak in each state. The general consensus is that social distancing will last for months until an effective vaccine is in place.

When Should I Wear a Mask?

In April, the Trump Administration recommended that everyone where a mask in public. This should be done *in addition to* and *not instead of* social distancing. Some people are still not wearing masks, citing the WHO and CDC's initial statements that masks would not stop of the spread of COVID-19 and thus need not be worn. *This has been revised* as more research regarding the infectiousness of the disease has surfaced. It is now the recommendation of both organizations that people wear masks whenever in public.

Contact Tracing[88]

The CDC has issued contact tracing guidelines to stop the spread of coronavirus. Tens of thousands of new public health workers have been enlisted and trained in contact tracing in recent months. In an interview with *WebMD,* Crystal Watson, senior scholar with the Johns Hopkins Center for Health Security, stated that contact tracing "is the best tool we have to manage this in an ongoing way to allow our economy to open up again." Watson has estimated that over 100,000 contact tracers will be needed in the U.S. to effectively stem the tide of the virus. That is a far cry from the currently trained 30,000 tracers, but the nation has expanded training at a rapid pace to meet this demand.

Contact tracing is a century-old public health tactic that involves isolation of a contaminated person and those with whom he or she came into contact. Because of the exponential increase in COVID-19 patients and the limited testing capacity, social isolation and lockdowns have been used to prevent spread. Now as the economy reopens and as testing supplies are more available, contact tracing may be a more viable approach. Early in the pandemic I spent 15 minutes in close contact with a patient removing his knee staples without appropriate PPE, and he was found to be COVID + the next day. There was no testing of asymptomatic staff at that time. In June, the situation was very different. One of the patients whom I tested resulted positive for COVID-19. Although I was wearing proper PPE during the visit, I was contacted as part of the tracing effort and tested promptly, thankfully found to be negative. One staff member was found to be positive and quickly quarantined—this is a paragon of effective contact tracing.

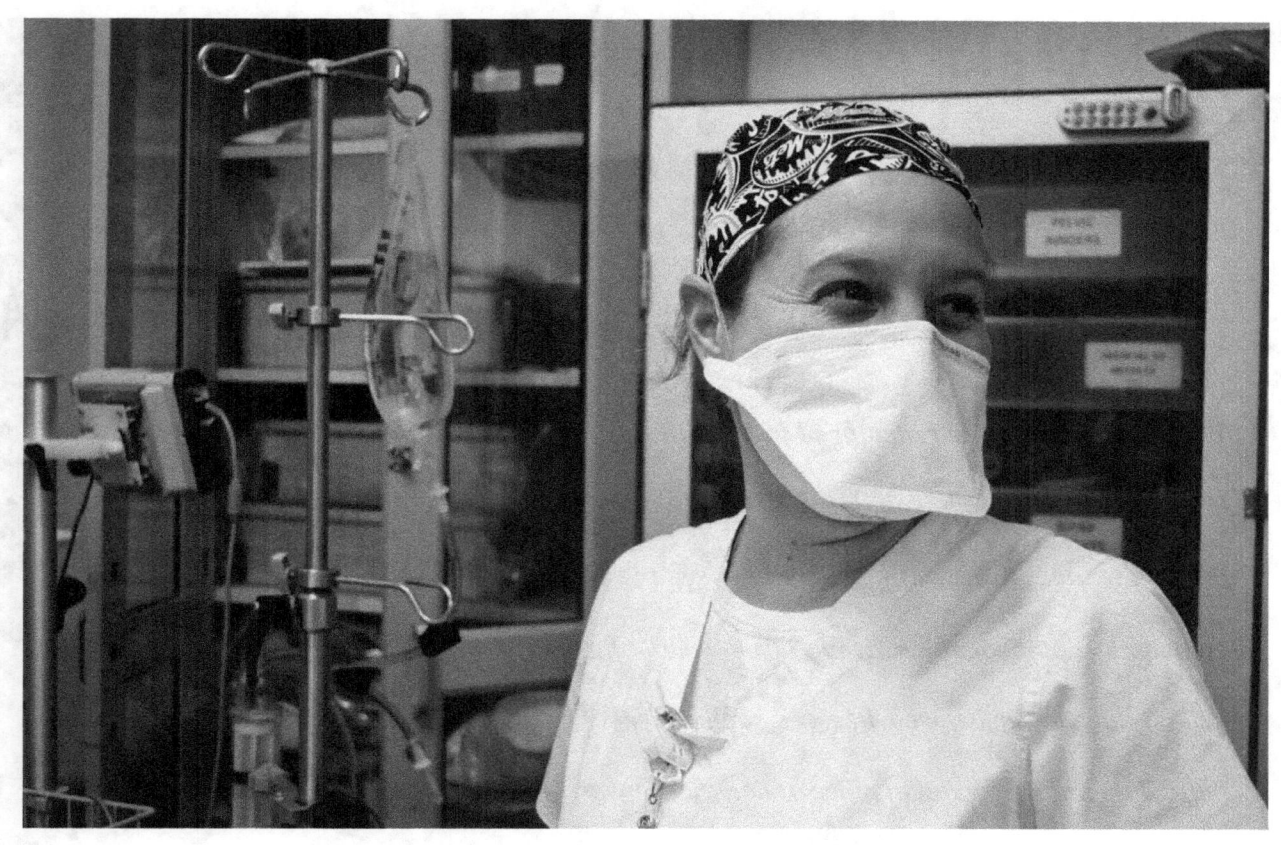

"Not everyone can do what we do. I'm proud of my ER team and how we have collaborated during this time."

-Diana Canzoneri, Registered Nurse, Emergency Department, NYC

Redeployed to Queens

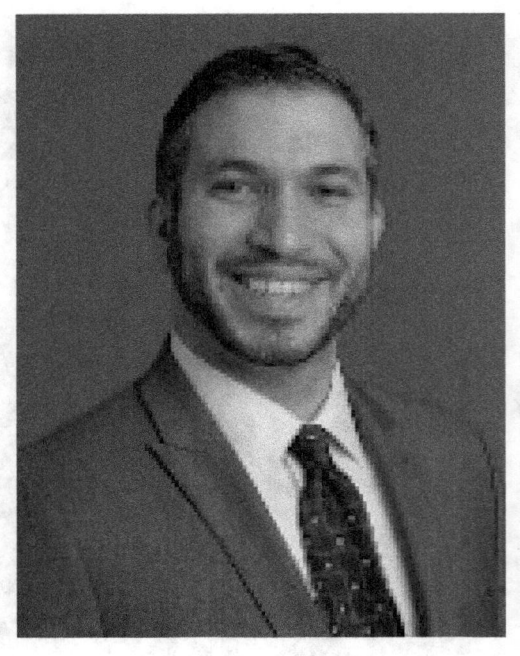

-Dr. Michael Prodromou, MD, Pulmonary Critical Care/ICU Attending at Mt. Sinai, NYC

What was it like to be redeployed to Mt. Sinai Queens—one of the hospitals most heavily impacted in the pandemic? *It was really touching to see the medical community come together during our moment of greatest need. I have never before witnessed such a level of camaraderie, bravery and willingness to help. I met a significant number of healthcare workers that were redeployed like myself and a few doctors who were flown in from Denver. One doctor had come to NY for vacation and then ended up volunteering with us in the hospital instead.*

Were there any patient experiences that most affected you? *As a physician, it is hard not to be concerned about your own health and safety when you routinely see suffering and pain. Normally, you ascribe patient's medical conditions to their advanced age, bad habits, or circumstance that is separate from your own. However, it was painfully obvious that no one is immune from COVID-19. I saw healthy people of my own age with severe infections and this was a sobering reality that we are all at risk of contracting the disease.*

Did many of your COVID patients die? *A significant number passed away. You couldn't tell who would die. I saw young people with no past medical history pass away, and 70 or 80-*

year-olds with a lot of medical issues do just fine. Of those that did die, they all looked fine on low amounts of oxygen initially but as time went on they would need other forms of ventilation including intubation. I couldn't tell you who would do well and who wouldn't do well the first time I saw them.

What was it like for family members who weren't able to be with their loved ones when they passed? *It was really tough. During my pre-COVID-19 ICU experience, family members could digest the idea of letting go by witnessing what the patient was going through, the medical care that they were receiving, and slowly come to terms with the fact that the patient was not getting better despite exhausting all medical efforts. In time, they would understand that their loved one may not be able to get better. That idea of letting go, and not allowing your family member to suffer unnecessarily is something that the family needs to understand in a step-wise fashion. It's an active process that occurs at the bedside. In the era of COVID-19, that crucial family experience was reduced to FaceTiming and Skyping, as family members were not allowed to come to the hospital, for obvious reasons. As a result, family members were making end-of-life decisions over the phone, and didn't get the closure they needed. I'm worried that they will not be able to heal from their loss because of this.*

What was it like for patients not to have family with them? *When you're a patient, any interaction with a loved one really helps. When you are deprived of that, you lose a little of your arsenal and your will to keep fighting. I think the death that COVID-19 patients experienced was one of the worst deaths someone could go through. I'm saying this from a* *humanistic point of view. Patients did not have the opportunity to interact with their families. They were unable to see emotion on their providers' faces as they were covered in PPE. They couldn't even see a smile from a nurse or doctor to help brighten their day because of the masks. They died alone. Since we were so saturated with patients, their bodies were placed in a temporary morgue. Thankfully this is changing more as things are opening up and the burden isn't as bad, but during the peak, it was terrible.*

Final thoughts? *It was an honor to serve, and I am sure that I have been forever changed by this experience, but I hope that we do not have to do it again. If we do have a second peak, the good thing is that we understand the disease better and will be more prepared with supplies. This was the first time we ever had to ration PPE and worry about ventilators and hospital beds to this extent. If this happens again, we will be better prepared.*

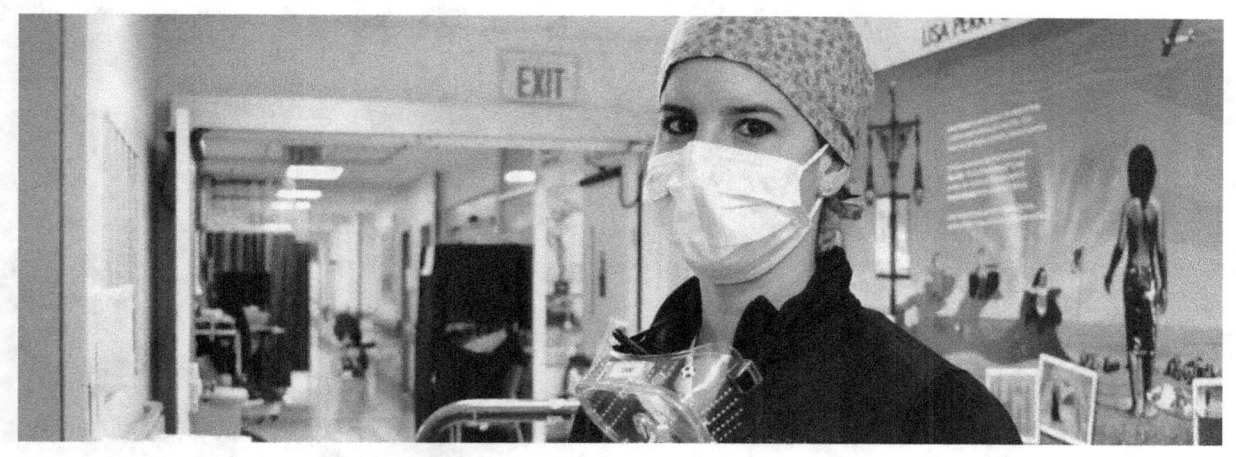

"It's a little different now. Walking to work I get this pit in my stomach. It's always been stressful, but never like this. But then I get to work and look around and see my coworkers, my team, I know I can do this with them by my side. They are the most brave, selfless, and resilient people I know. We may all be a little scared right now, but we've got each other and we've got this."

-Danielle Ruthberg, Registered Nurse, Emergency Department, NYC

Working on the Front Lines

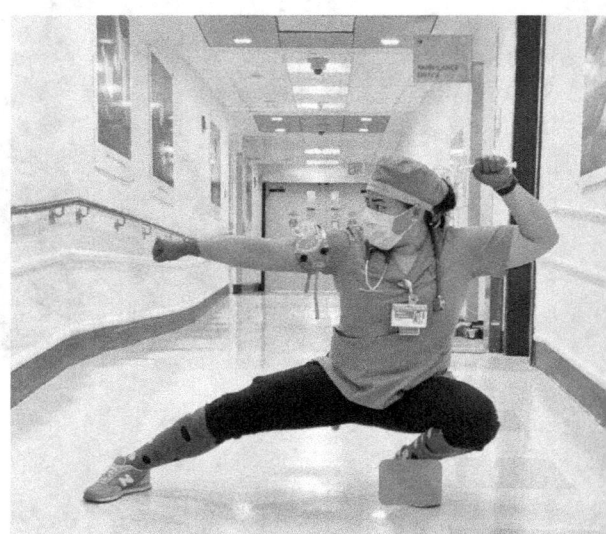

-Camille Culbengan, Registered Nurse, Pediatric Emergency Department, NYC

Originally Published on Health Matters

I am not only proud, I am honored to be on the front lines. When we heard the outcry of our adult teammates, we wanted to help them and be there in solidarity.

It's different when you just hear about the pandemic being grim and tragic, but now that it's in my home and right in front of me, it affects me much differently. One of the biggest challenges I've faced occurred was when I was working overtime in the adult ED. I was walking in the hallway grabbing supplies, and there was a patient calling out for a nurse, so I stopped by. She said, "Nurse, I am scared. I'm so scared that I'm going to die alone."

I held her hand and I told her, "It's OK to be scared. We're all scared, but you're not alone. I'm here with you." This patient was so grateful that I took the time out to talk to her, but to see the fear and suffering in her eyes really affected me. Once I finished speaking to her, I had to step away and cry because that's when it really hit home. All you can do is just be there for the patient. You see your co-workers who are overwhelmed; you see very sick patients. It's very heartbreaking, but we push through together as a team and we're there for each other, and we're going to fight this. We will get through this.

CHAPTER 10: MEDICAL COMPLICATIONS OF COVID-19

"Miner had seen influenza often. He diagnosed the disease as influenza. But he had never seen influenza like this. This was violent, rapid in its progress through the body, and sometimes lethal. This influenza killed. Soon dozens of his patients—the strongest, the healthiest, the most robust people in the country—were being struck down as suddenly as if they had been shot."

-John M. Barry in *The Great Influenza*

I remember the first time I had to tell a patient the results of her COVID-19 test. People are understandably terrified of acquiring COVID-19. Not only can the disease be life-threatening, but even those who survive can have impairments that require prolonged rehabilitation and that impact their daily activities and ability to work. In this chapter, I discuss COVID-19 symptoms and some of the severe complications we see with the disease.

Symptoms

Symptoms of COVID-19 usually manifest between 2 and 14 days after exposure to the virus. Patients may experience cough, shortness of breath, fever, chills, body ache, sore throat, diarrhea, and lack of taste and smell. Severe cases can cause massive alveolar damage and progressive respiratory failure that can lead to death[14,15,16]. Symptom duration can range from less than a day to months.

Complications

About one in six people suffer medical complications from COVID-19[113], usually due to cytokine storm—an intense inflammatory response to the viral pathogen. Medical complications include liver and kidney injury, septic shock, and COVID coagulopathy--an increase in hypercoagulable state that can lead to clots and strokes. An increase in inflammatory markers such as CRP, ESR, and D-Dimer level have been seen in COVID-19 patients, and are often used to track the severity of the disease process.

Respiratory Complications

Severe respiratory complications that can result from COVID-19 include pneumonia, bronchitis, and ARDS. Forty percent of patients with severe cases of COVID-19 develop acute respiratory distress syndrome (ARDS) and 50% of those patients die from the disease. The median time to intubation reported by hospitals is 11 days. Of those intubated, 75-85%

eventually succumb to the disease. Those who survive may have significant impairments such as encephalopathy and critical illness neuropathy and myopathy. Recent findings show that even people with asymptomatic or mild cases have evidence of lung compromise on imaging.

Kidney/Liver damage

Many intubated COVID-19 patients are requiring dialysis due to kidney failure. The kidney plays an essential role in eliminating waste, balancing electrolytes, and controlling blood pressure, and end-stage-renal failure can rapidly lead to death without life-saving dialysis. COVID-19 appears to cause direct damage to the kidney and liver, and associated hypoxia may also cause secondary damage. According to nephrologist, Dr. Rebecca Babayev, patients who develop kidney failure usually have poor outcomes. But those who survive are likely to recover renal function completely.

Neurological Impact

Every infection can trigger stroke, because of the increase in blood pressure and inflammatory markers. However, early on it was identified that COVID-19 patients are at higher than usual risk for developing clots and strokes. This is thought to be due to the hypercoagulable state discussed above. Superinfection with bacterial pathogens may also result in septic embolization. Even young patients were at high risk of this devastating complication. COVID-19 patients with elevated D-Dimer levels are being treated with high dose anticoagulation, such as used to treat acute deep vein thromboses (DVTs) and atrial fibrillation and to prevent stroke. Anticoagulation can increase bleeding risk, but the risks of clots and stroke are so high in these patients that in most cases the benefits of anticoagulation outweighs the costs.

Post-delirium extubation is common in non-COVID patients as well, but COVID patients are being intubated for much longer durations than typical, and thus suffering from prolonged neurological sequela and musculoskeletal wasting. Encephalopathy is impaired cognition due to disruption to the brain. In COVID-19, this is suspected to be caused by anoxic brain injury, or a lack of oxygen due to the disease, or a post-viral autoimmune response. In the TBI unit, I saw some severe, cases of encephalopathy in COVID-19 patients who were status post intubation—some resolved and some did not. Critical illness neuropathy and myopathy describe muscle weakness and nerve damage associated with severe sickness and prolonged hospital stay. These conditions require prolonged rehabilitation to improve patients' function and to help them to return to work and their prior quality of life. Thus, surviving COVID-19 is not enough; one also must survive its sequela.

Can COVID-19 Affect Pregnancy/Lactation?

The 1918 Spanish Influenza affected pregnant women at alarming rates. Even women who survived often lost their babies. Thankfully, there is absolutely no data to suggest that pregnant women are at greater risk from COVID-19[70]. That being said, pregnant women are at a higher risk for respiratory illness, and this can result in dangerous outcomes for both mother and child[70]. Pregnant women should practice social distancing and frequent handwashing as all others should.

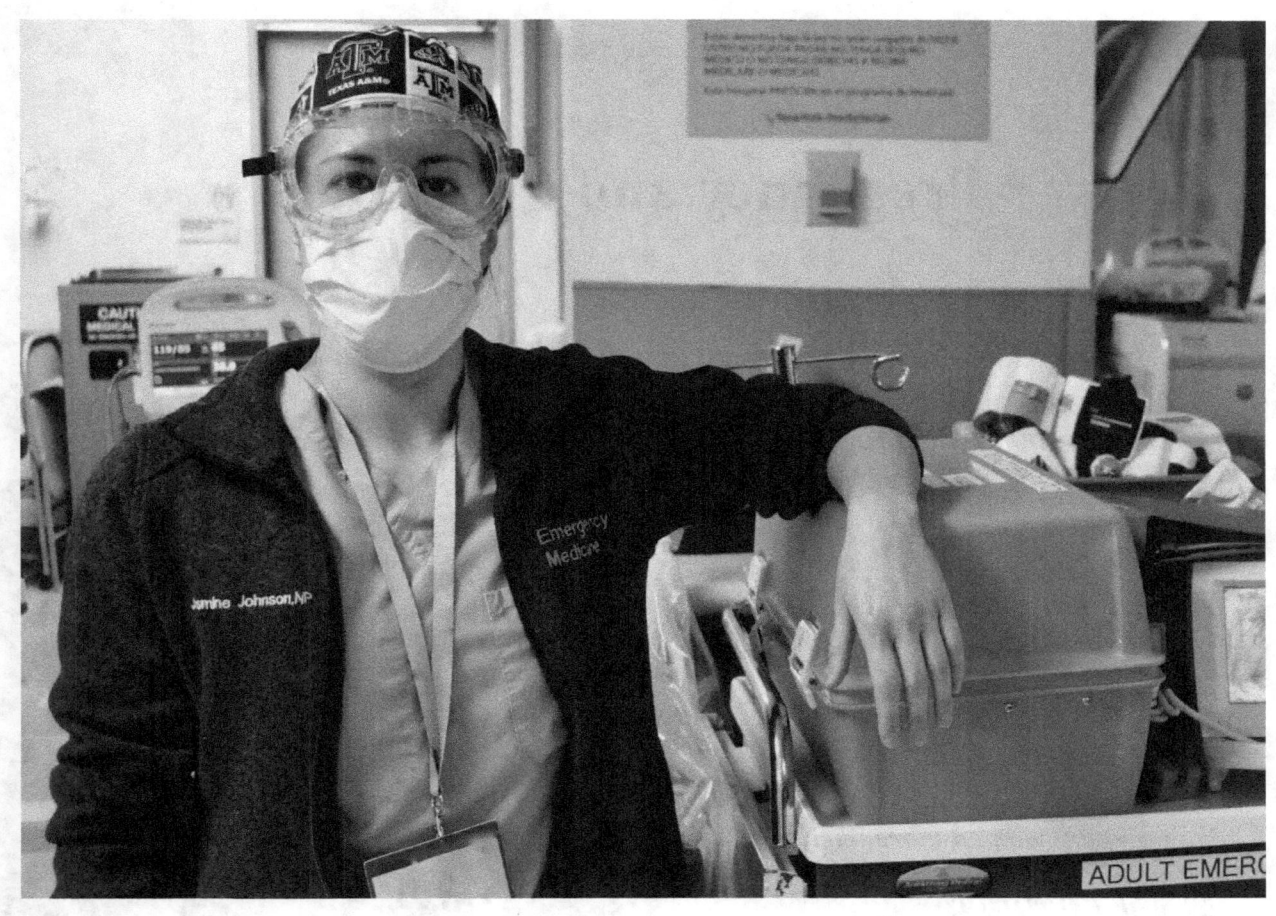

"Although this experience has been physically and mentally draining, I feel honored to be able to be here, at this hospital, in this city, during one of the biggest events of our lifetimes, fighting for others."

-Jasmine Johnson, Nurse Practitioner, Emergency Department, NYC

Pregnancy and COVID-19

- Dr. Laura Riley, MD, Department of Obstetrics and Gynecology, NYC

Original interview by Alyssa Sunkin-Strube and Jordan Lite

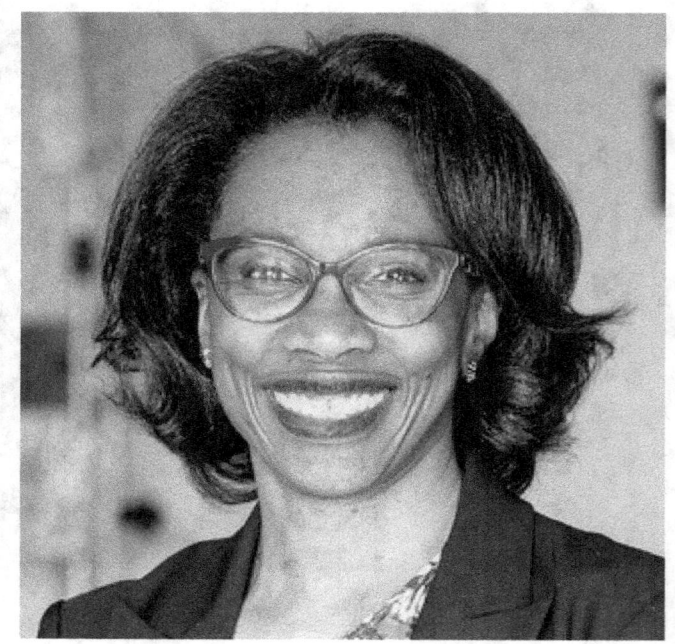

Are pregnant women more likely to become sick with COVID-19?

There is limited data on pregnant women who have been infected with COVID-19, the disease caused by the new coronavirus. This limited data suggests that pregnant women are no more likely to develop serious symptoms than others.

How can pregnant women protect themselves and their babies?

Pregnant women should protect themselves as everyone else in the general public should, and follow the CDC's recommendations.

• Wash your hands often with soap and water for at least 20 seconds or use an alcohol-based *hand sanitizer that contains 60% to 95% alcohol.*

- *Avoid touching your eyes, nose, and mouth with unwashed hands.*

- *Avoid close contact with anyone sick.*

- *Stay home when you are sick.*

- *Cover your cough or sneeze with a tissue, and then throw the tissue in the trash and wash your hands for 20 seconds. If you do not have a tissue, cough or sneeze into your elbow, rather than into your hands.*

- *Clean and disinfect frequently touched objects and surfaces.*

It's also really important to practice **social distancing**, *staying at least 6 feet away from people when out in public and avoiding social gatherings.*

How can I boost my immunity while pregnant? Should I be working out?

The best thing is to rely on rest, a good diet, vitamin C, and maybe even **meditation**. *There is no one pill. It's important to continue your physical activity. This is going to help with the natural* **anxiety** *that comes with this situation.*

Does COVID-19 cause pregnancy complications or birth defects?

The data available suggests that a COVID-19 infection does not cause birth defects. It may cause a slight increase in the risk of preterm birth, but this is unclear. Researchers are actively studying whether COVID-19 can be passed to babies in utero.

What should I do if I'm experiencing flu or COVID-19 symptoms?

If you develop **flu-like symptom**s *while you're pregnant, it's important that you call your* *obstetrician or midwife. The flu is still circulating, and you may have the flu. With pregnancy, we know that influenza can be very serious, and we would treat you with antiviral medications. COVID-19 is a possibility, so it's important to tell your provider before you come to the hospital or doctor's office so we can be prepared and assess whether a* **virtual visit** *or an in-person evaluation is needed. Pregnant women should avoid seeking care at an emergency department whenever possible. Your obstetrician or midwife is the most qualified expert to help you.*

Can any of my prenatal appointments be virtual?

In general, women have between 12 and 14 visits overall during a routine pregnancy, and I think it's clear that you don't need all 14 to still have good prenatal care. Which visit can be avoided or which visit can be replaced with a video visit really depends on your pregnancy. The best thing to do is call your provider and ask their opinion. If you are healthy and not experiencing complications, you may be able to transition several prenatal appointments to video visits.

Can I be tested for COVID-19 if I'm pregnant?

Our hospital is currently testing patients in the hospital and pregnant patients who are coming in to deliver a baby, as well as a few other patient populations. If you have been exposed to COVID-19 or are experiencing symptoms, it's important that you call and let us know you are concerned about possible exposure. If you are advised to visit a healthcare provider, you will be directed to use a mask throughout your visit and coordinate your visit time to minimize exposure to others.

Can I breastfeed if I have COVID-19 or suspect that I do?

You can breastfeed your baby. There is no data that shows the virus is in breastmilk. But take precautions to avoid spreading it to your infant, including washing your hands before touching your baby and wearing a face mask.

Treating Renal Failure from COVID-19

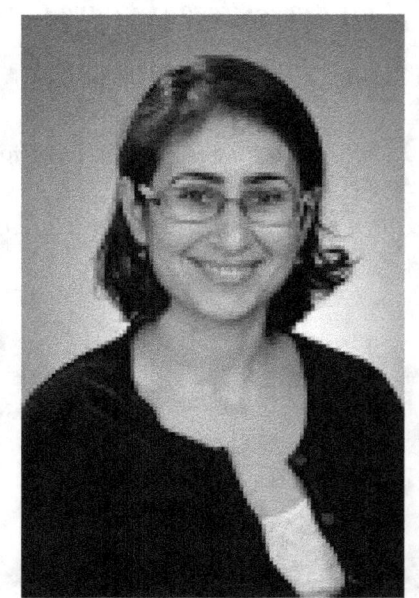

—Dr. Revekka Babayev, MD, Nephrologist, CT

What was it like to work as a nephrologist during the COVID-19 pandemic? One of the main challenges for my colleagues working in New York was resource allocation. There were not enough dialysis nurses or even dialysis machines at one point. For us, we were lucky to have enough nurses but due to limitations of equipment, some dialysis patients were receiving treatments twice a week instead of three times or some patients who required continues replacement therapies were getting them for 12hours on, 12 hours off. For my colleagues at CUMC and Montefiore who were the hardest hit, they had it harder and had to give them just enough to get by based on what was available.

For me there were two main challenges. One was working with the unknown. There are patients in multi-organ failure requiring dialysis. Initially we were trying to keep lungs dryer but people were crashing. We started from scratch and instead tried to keep people a little more positive. We added anticoagulation to their dialysis machines to reduce clotting. There were new changes every day. You felt like you were shooting in the dark a lot of the time. It's so tough when you see a lot of patients not make it. Stamford is a community hospital and ECMO was not available. Other institutions were not accepting patients because *they were overwhelmed. We are used to giving the best care possible without thought to limited resources, and it is so difficult to deny patients potentially life-saving treatment.*

As consultants, we have been offering televisits for COVID+ patients so as not to waste limited PPE. I was putting patients on dialysis without ever talking to them face to face. It was depersonalizing. Some of my colleagues were afraid to round in the hospital and risk exposure to the virus. Personally, I couldn't round remotely. I needed to provide emotional support to my team.

Did many vented patients develop renal failure? *About twenty percent of vented patients developed acute kidney injury. Of those that developed renal failure, 2/3 did not make it. Once you were vented and on dialysis outcomes are really poor.*

Did patients experience kidney injury directly from the virus or from related hypoxia? *Data so far suggests the mechanism of injury is both the direct acute tubular injury from the virus as well as the body's cytokine storm in reaction to the disease. A lot of our ICU patients are also hypotensive, and thus have further ischemic insults from low blood pressures.*

Does renal failure usually resolve? *In those patients who have survived and were able to avoid other setbacks almost all recovered renal function.*

Final thoughts? *There has been a lot of talk about African Americans and Hispanics being at higher risk of renal failure from COVID-19. Data is emerging as to whether higher levels of the APOE1 allele may be related to higher rates of kidney failure in this population.*

My boys, age 7 and 11 are legitimately scared for me. I come home and nobody touches me until I shower and scrub everything down. You don't want to get your family sick but you also don't want to isolate from them. You just have to be as careful as possible so you can be comfortable with your family. It's been an adventure.

CHAPTER 11:

TREATMENTS FOR COVID-19

"What did bother him was the need to abandon good science. To succeed in preparing either a vaccine or a serum, he would have to make a series of guesses based on at best inconclusive results, and each guess would have to be right."

–John M. Barry in *The Great Influenza*

The first step in management of COVID-19 includes immediate isolation to prevent spread. Most patients are able to self-quarantine at home and do not need to go to the emergency room. Staying at home is actually recommended to limit the spread of the virus. If feasible, patients can have a virtual care visit or phone call with their primary care physicians to discuss their symptoms and a plan of care. NY State made such visits free for its residents. NY also supplied self-test kits for people to self-administer in their homes. If patients are with respiratory distress and oxygen desaturation, they may require hospital admission for supplemental oxygen. They may first receive a nasal cannula—a 2-pronged device placed in the nostrils that can deliver up to 6L of oxygen. If difficulty breathing persists, they may be transitioned to a non-rebreather—a facemask that can provide a higher percentage of oxygen—or a BiPAP machine, a ventilator that provides positive airway pressure to the lungs through a facemask.

If respiratory distress and oxygen desaturation continue despite supplemental oxygen, patients may require intubation and mechanical ventilation. Intubation greatly increases the chance of death; approximately 75-85% of COVID-19 patients who are intubated ultimately die. Pre-COVID-19, patients were often intubated for persistent oxygen saturation lower than 85%, and this policy was adopted early in the pandemic. But soon it became clear that those being intubated did not have better outcomes, and the policy was quickly re-adjusted. As Dr. Anthony DeVivo describes, a subset of COVID-19 patients were referred to as "happy hypoxics" because despite scarily low oxygen saturations, they were able to converse and sometimes appeared comfortable and happy.

There has been much attention to the use of proning for COVID-19 patients[39]. Proning is positioning the patients flat on their stomachs in a "prone" position, allowing greater oxygen of their lungs by gravity, because there is a larger volume of tissue in the back of the lungs[39]. This causes abnormal fluids and secretions that form in response to COVID-19 to accumulate in the front of the lung and keep the back of the lungs aerated[39]. The technique is typically used for influenza patients that have ARDS, and imaging of COVID-19 patients' lungs shows bilateral patchy infiltrates very similar to those found in ARDS. A 2013 *New England Journal of Medicine* article describes how early proning during ARDS treatment decreases mortality. Proning requires no equipment, though special proning beds are available, and many frontline providers have identified it as one of the most effective tools they have against the virus. A *Times* article written by a patient's husband describes how his wife was told she had only a couple of hours left to live due to COVID-19, but she recovered after being proned[39]. The United Kingdom Intensive Care Society recommends that proning be used early in treatment, prior to the need for intensive care to reduce the need for invasive ventilation and death[39]. Rush University Medical Center is currently conducting a clinical trial to assess the value of proning for patients with mild to moderate symptoms who require supplemental oxygen[39]. Proning is not appropriate for certain populations, such as pregnant women, the morbidly obese, or those with facial injuries[39].

Medications

There are currently no medications approved by the Food and Drug Administration for the treatment of COVID-19[34]. It takes an exorbitant amount of time for drugs to be tested and deemed effective and safe for use in humans. Repurposing of existing clinical drugs has been a popular option in the pandemic since drugs that have already been vetted would not need to undergo as extensive of a review process[34].

At the University of Minnesota Medical Center, Dr. Susan Line is conducting an international clinical trial on the effects of remdesivir, an antiviral medication that thus far seems to be the most effective treatment for severe cases of COVID-19. Dr. Klines' current findings are that patients who receive remdesivir recover in an average of 11 days as opposed to 15 days for those who do not receive the drug. Her results are preliminary and have not yet been published, reviewed, and replicated, but given the dire need for treatments, the NIH has authorized the use of remdesivir on an emergency basis.

Early studies noted mild efficacy of hydroxychloroquine (Plaquenil) and azithromycin, and in response, on March 28th the FDA allowed release of the nation's stockpile of these agents for emergency use [33,34]. However, the early studies were small and with short follow up and did not assess side effects[33]. More recent larger studies have failed to prove their efficacy. These drugs also have significant side effects for certain patients.

Hydroxychloroquine is typically used to treat malaria, lupus, and rheumatoid arthritis through immunosuppression[32]. Thus, it has been speculated to have benefit in COVID-19 by suppressing the dangerous and organ-damaging cytokine storm that results as patients mount an immune response to the virus[32]. Azithromycin is an antibiotic commonly used for the treatment of pneumonia. While earlier studies noted mild efficacy of these agents, larger studies have not replicated these findings. A recent study in France found that 600mg of daily hydroxychloroquine (more than we typically administer) does not help to reduce ICU admission rate or mortality, though it may provide some symptomatic relief. The VA conducted a study evaluating 368 patients who received placebo or hydroxychloroquine alone or with azithromycin. It found no benefit from the drug and a higher death rate for patients who received hydroxychloroquine[67,69]. Hydroxychloroquine can also increase the qTC interval, which can lead to life-threatening arrhythmias. Another fear voiced regarding its overuse was that there would be a lack of hydroxychloroquine to treat the diseases for which it is conventionally used and considered an important therapeutic agent. Hydroxychloroquine has also gained national attention from President Trump, who has shared that he has been using Hydroxychloroquine prophylactically as per his physician's recommendations[68]. He has been criticized for promoting a drug that has not been rigorously scientifically proven to have benefit against the disease.

A JAMA retrospective cohort study of 1,438 patients did not show reduced mortality from COVID-19 after treatment with either hydroxychloroquine alone or in combination with azithromycin[33]. In April, nearly all our patients were receiving a combination of hydroxychloroquine and azithromycin despite minimal evidence in support of these treatments. As more robust studies continued to show no change in mortality, there appeared to be a reduction in their use, but this decision was not always accepted by patients and their family members. Dr. Berg, a critical care pulmonologist at Good Samaritan Hospital in Rockland County, recalls how he has been challenged by patients' family members regarding why their loved ones were not receiving hydroxychloroquine. His explanation that the medication was contraindicated given his patients' prolonged qTC intervals was often met with resistance. Understandably, patients want to advocate for their family members and ensure they are receiving the best care possible. As they have sworn in the Hippocratic Oath, healthcare providers want to "do no harm" and are hesitant to prescribe unproven medications that may hurt more than help according to available literature. On June 18th, the WHO discontinued its trial of hydroxyquinolone, citing lack of beneficiary evidence for the medication[130].

Tocilizumab is a monoclonal antibody that is used as an immunosuppressant for its high affinity in binding to the IL-6 receptor[37]. Xu et al showed efficacy of tocilizumab in treating patients with severe disease[38]. As per Dr. Berg, tocilizumab comes with severe side effects—he estimates that there is a 20% chance of bacterial sepsis in patients who receive this drug.

Neutralizing Antibodies[112]

One June 1st, pharmaceutical giant Eli Lilly started the first trials to develop monoclonal antibodies to bind to the COVID-19 antigen. Monoclonal antibodies are often used to treat cancer and autoimmune disease. One week after initiation of trials. Eli Lilly reported that it has two potential targets in phase 1 trials, which test the safety and tolerability of the drug in a small group of health participants. The agents bind to different epitopes of the COVID-19 spike proteins, so the company plans to use both in a cocktail approach against the disease. Eli Lilly's chief scientist has announced that the treatment could be available as early as September[126].

Dexamethasone

Steroids are often used to treat severe inflammation, though at the risk of immunosuppression. In the case of COVID-19 where a hyper-immune response can be lethal, a recent British study shows that the commonly prescribed steroid dexamethasone may reduce death by 1/3 for those on ventilators and 1/5 for those on other forms of oxygen supplementation[124]. Researchers estimate that if the drug had been used early in treatment, up to 5,000 British lives would have been saved. The British study has yet to be released.

Currently the NIH and academic institutions are conducting well-powered randomized control trials to provide more accurate information regarding the efficacy of these and other possible therapeutics.

Dietary Supplements

One study also found that Vitamin D deficiency may be associated with higher rates of mortality due to COVID-19[35]. The study individuals who lived in countries with lower levels of vitamin D exposure, such as Spain and Italy, had higher rates of mortality. Vitamin D is one of the most commonly deficient vitamins, as it is not as available in foods. Instead, high levels of Vitamin D can be obtained by sunlight exposure. As people spend more time inside and wear sunscreen when they venture into the hot summer rays, their absorption of Vitamin D will decrease. It is currently recommended that women over the age of 65 be tested for Vitamin D deficiency given their increased risk of osteoporosis post-menopause, and the important role of Vitamin D in the absorption of calcium, essential for building strong bones. Vitamin D toxicity is relatively rare so it is safe for most people to consume a small daily dose, and most COVID-19 patients are currently receiving Vitamin D supplementation.

Another vitamin that has received press for its immune- stimulating effects is Vitamin C, ascorbic acid[36]. Research has found that vitamin C can help in the development and maturation of T lymphocytes that are essential in mounting a cellular immune response[36].

Convalescent Plasma

The use of convalescent plasma that contains antibodies from patients who have recovered from COVID-19 has shown anecdotal success, but clinical trials investigating its efficacy are still needed and it is not an FDA approved treatment[37]. It can currently be provided through a clinical research trial or on an emergency basis if requested by a physician for a patient with severe or life-threatening symptoms[37]. The FDA defines severe symptoms as one or more of the following: respiratory frequency $\geq$ 30/min, blood oxygen saturation $\leq$ 93%, partial pressure of arterial oxygen to fraction of inspired oxygen ratio < 300, and lung infiltrates > 50% within 24 to 48 hours[37]. Life-threatening disease is characterized by at least one of the following: respiratory failure, septic shock, multiple organ dysfunction or failure[37].

In order to donate, patients must be 14 days free of COVID symptoms[37]. They need not have a negative test[37]. Convalescent plasma has been used in past outbreaks, such as the 2002 SARS-CoV1 and 2013 MERS-CoV epidemics and the 2009 H1N1 influenza pandemic.

Vaccine

The most definitive treatment for COVID-19, and what we are all anxious for, is a vaccine. Experts say it may take over a year for a COVID-19 vaccine to be developed. China is a frontrunner in producing coronavirus vaccines, and Chinese president Xi Jinping has pledged to make any effective vaccine widely available to all countries[73]. As of May, China has 5 vaccines in clinical trials and more than 2,000 people enrolled in phase II trials[73], which test the safety and efficacy of a drug or vaccine in a larger population of humans once it has already been shown to be safe in a smaller population Phase I trial. Before a vaccine can reach the masses, it must then pass a much larger randomized control Phase III trial in which efficacy is compared between patients who received and did not receive the disease in a region where the pandemic is rampant[73].

As per infectious diseases specialist Dr. Lynda Streett, it is possible that multiple vaccines will be launched at the same time given the worldwide race to produce one. On July 16th, the U.S. Department of Health and Safety announced that a COVID-19 vaccine would be free for patients at highest risk for COVID-19 who could not otherwise afford it[130]. Even once a vaccine is available, many people will be afraid to receive it until thorough safety testing data is available.

> **When will a vaccine be available?**
>
> Director of the CDC Infectious Diseases Department, Dr. Anthony S. Fauci, has said he is hopeful that a vaccine will be available in late 2020 to early 2021.

Rehabilitation

As a physiatrist, I would be remiss to exclude a section on rehabilitation, an essential but often unspoken part of recovery for many COVID patients who are severely debilitated after prolonged hospital stays and intubation. Critical illness myopathy is rampant in these patients, as young adults lose approximately 1% of muscle mass for every day on bed rest; the elderly are at risk for a 5% daily loss due to decreased levels of growth hormone[118]. In COVID-19 patients we also saw some severe cases of encephalopathy and critical illness neuropathy on top of the need for cardiopulmonary rehabilitation. At the large free-standing rehabilitation hospital where I worked, we were fortunate to have enough space to devote a whole rehabilitation floor to COVID + patients, allowing them to receive therapy in the gym as per usual protocol. Our hospitals have 16 and 22 beds respectively, so COVID-19 patients had to receive therapy in their rooms to prevent spread as is the case for all patients on droplet precautions. In the early days of the pandemic, when rehabilitation facilities at other New York hospitals shut down, our rehabilitation centers expanded to accept traumatic brain and spinal cord injury patients. Additional rehabilitation and recovery wings were also opened as consults for COVID-19 patients soared. Many required rehabilitation for shorter stays than our typical patients, and were able to be discharged home with oxygen after a few days. Others required prolonged rehabilitation stays and had residual cognitive deficits once they were discharged home.

Pediatric to Adult ED

-Dr. Anju Wagh, MD, Pediatric Emergency Medicine Physician, NYC

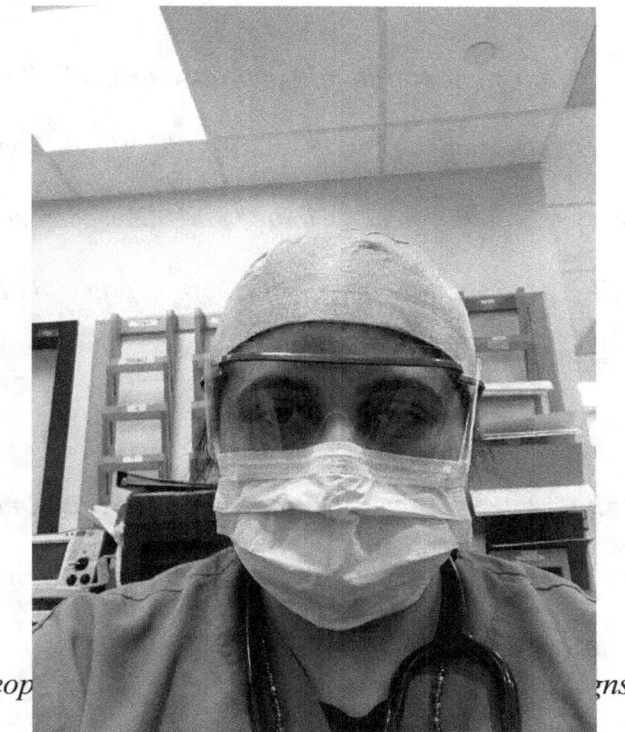

What was it like to work in the adult ED during the peak of the pandemic? A bunch of us volunteered to work in the adult ED, where they were so short of people. I walked around, changed oxygen tanks, made sure people's vital signs were stable. If someone was not ok, I would alert their attendings. I'm one of the old-timers so I was able to put in IVs and draw labs. I was willing to help with anything that was needed.

Did you treat any patients with pediatric multi-inflammatory syndrome? We started seeing them in the last week of April. By then we were the central hospital so we were seeing a fair number.

What symptoms did they have? The most common symptom was a high fever. Also, conjunctivitis, rash, mucositis. Many had symptoms of myositis (inflammation of the heart, measured by increased markers in the blood).

Is this similar to Kawasaki disease?

It's not Kawasaki exactly, as most of these patients did not have carotid artery involvement.

Were most patients admitted or discharged? *Most of them were admitted. Some were in the ICU, they needed pressure support for shock. Some were on the regular floor for monitoring. Very few died—those who died had other comorbidities. Most patients responded very well to IVIG, steroids, and anakinra. There was eventually an IVIG shortage because 10-15 patients per day were requiring it.*

What patient experiences most affected you? *In the adult ED, they were all alone. They were so sick and had nobody there. At least children were allowed one caretaker during the pandemic.*

What would you like people to know about COVID-19? *I think physicians were emotionally drained from seeing so much suffering and from the stress of the uncertainty. Some of us felt that we didn't do enough and there was definitely an element of guilt.*

Final thoughts? *Where were the other kids? Volumes of pediatric ER visits were down by 50-60% or more. Kids are not in school and thus not exposed to infection. They are not doing sports, and thus not getting injured. Many adult EDs are also experiencing a decreased in non-COVID adult visits across the country.*

Are you concerned that many children are missing their vaccinations? *There is a concern when I speak to pediatricians because so many vaccinations have been delayed. I think it depends on how long things will be affected. Already there is an increasing amount of anti-vaxxers and as a result, reduced rates of herd immunity.*

Getting COVID-19

-Emily Jackson, Nursing Director in the Division of Medicine and Neurosciences, NYC

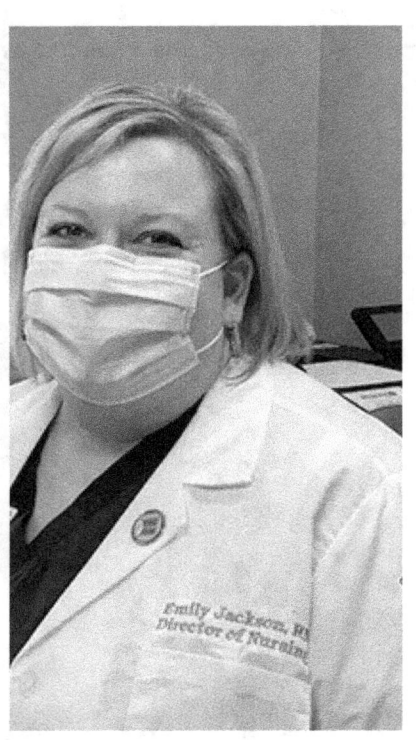

Originally Published on HealthMatters

It started as a cough and a low-grade fever, and it soon progressed to chills and body aches. There were two or three days when I was scared, not knowing if it would progress to worsening symptoms. But by the fourth day, I started feeling better, which was a huge relief. Honestly, when my test came back positive for COVID-19, I was a bit relieved. At that point, I was beginning to feel better, and I knew I was going to be OK. Still, I was shocked at how tired and lethargic I was for some time afterward. The shortness of breath and fatigue lasted for a couple of weeks, but I was on the mend.

Then, like most people in quarantine, I started to get bored and restless. Mainly I just wanted to return to work to support my team. As a director of nursing, my job is to take care of front-line staff and make sure they have the supplies and support they need to take the best possible care of our patients. I stayed in touch with my team by phone and email and could not wait to get back to work, knowing that I could be more effective in the hospital. However, it was important to me to not infect anyone else and follow the quarantine timeline.

I now feel completely recovered, and I'm back to my baseline energy levels. If I have one message to share, it is this: If you do get sick, take the time to rest and recover. Do not be discouraged if it takes longer to feel better after this illness than any other time you've been sick. This is a new virus to humans, and your body is figuring out how to handle it. Rest and allow yourself the time to get better. If you do end up needing the hospital's services, we are here to take amazing care of you and will do our best to get you back home safely!

CHAPTER 12: COVID-19 AND CHILDREN

"I am a mom. I am a wife. I am a daughter. I am a sister. I am an Emergency Medicine PA. I come in each night to help those in need, and I try to do it with a smile under my mask. I lean on my family. I trust in my coworkers. We will get through this together."

-Jennine McAuley, Emergency Medicine Physician's Assistant

"Mama, why do you have to go to work when there is Coronavirus?" My 4-year-old son Riaan has grown up surrounded by my medical books as I studied through medical school, intern year, and residency and is fascinated by medicine. His preschool has closed due to COVID-19, as have his sports and karate classes. He sees his daddy working from home and is saddened that I will still be going to work. My husband bought him a book called "Viruses vs. Bacteria" and he understands that viruses invade the body, replicate, cause symptoms, and can infect other people, and we explain that mama still has patients to care for despite the coronavirus. Even my 18-month-old daughter Risa, who in her youthful innocence is blissfully unaware that we are living in a pandemic, always reminds me before we leave the house, "Mama, mask, wear."

One of the few positives of COVID-19 is that it generally does not cause severe disease in children[78], unlike influenza. Proposed reasons for children's lack of symptoms is that have not yet developed mature receptors for the virus to bind, or that they do not mount a severe "cytokine storm" response[78]. However, they can still be infected and may be more infectious than adults. They can thus be dangerous vectors since it is often difficult for them to keep their masks on and to keep away from other people and animals. Not to mention their desire to touch everything and for infants, taste everything!

Nevertheless, there have been cases in children with a 0.5% mortality rate. To put in perspective, this is half the 1.1% mortality rate of dying in a car accident. However, any death of a child is catastrophic. This is one of the reasons the 1918 pandemic, which affected children at an alarming rate, was so horrific.

School Closures

The pandemic has upended the education system with children around the country schooling from home to protect our youth, the teachers who educate them, and other school staff. Many schools will remain closed through the school year, and parents find themselves homeschooling their children through their Zoom and iPad mediated curriculums while simultaneously working from home. In some areas, the online education system is rife with problems. Rural districts have problem with internet access, kids must be highly motivated to keep up with their Zoom classes and coursework, and they are not as easily able to ask for teachers' help. Prolonged screen time and lack of in-person social interaction is not healthy, especially for our youngest students. I asked a couple of our neighborhood boys how they felt about school from home. One answered that he loved it, he had the chance to play video games all day! The other said he couldn't wait to go back as he was missing his friends. Almost every parent I spoke to is disenchanted if not overwhelmed by home schooling and can't wait for their children to return to school. If we didn't realize what heroes our teachers are, we certainly appreciate them now! It is possible that when schools do reopen there will be social distancing rules in place and children will be required to wear masks. School may also have separate hours for different children to limit the number of students in the school, for example, alternate day classes or morning and evening sessions.

In order to help healthcare workers get to work, some hospitals provided childcare for their employees. My son was able to go to Vivvi, an early childhood education center in the city where he received exceptional care and was in a class of only three students. NYC also tried to provide childcare for children of essential workers, and some caretakers volunteered to care for children in their own homes.

There have also been changes at the University level, with colleges closing their doors and sending their students home early. Many may continue to stay closed through the fall[22]. The largest 4- year college system, the California State School System, declared in May that they would not have in-person instruction in the fall[23]. The scholastic aptitude test (SAT) was waived as a requirement by many universities given students' disrupted school years. It is unclear whether this will be a temporary or more long-term change.

Pediatric Multisystem Inflammatory Syndrome

There have been cases of a Kawasaki-like post-viral syndrome in children, now called Pediatric Multisystem Inflammatory Syndrome, where children develop red tongue, high fevers, and a rash. This is a *reaction* to COVID-19, but not COVID itself. These children have been found to have positive COVID-19 antibodies in their blood. About 100 such cases were reported in NY state as of May 13th, and this number is likely a significant underestimate. My colleague suffered a scare in early April when her 15-month-old daughter developed symptoms of high fever and rash. This was before NY state had publicized the Kawasaki cases and we were worried that her daughter may be experiencing symptoms of COVID-19, but she and her family tested negative. Thankfully her daughter recovered quickly and most cases of Kawasaki self-resolve, but there have been 5 devastating deaths of young children from this syndrome in NY.

Decrease in Child Vaccination

As parents fear to take their children outside of their homes, especially to healthcare facilities, children are missing their recommended vaccinations. According to the Michigan Care Registry, vaccination coverage declined in all age cohorts, except for the first Hepatitis B vaccine that is administered at birth[87]. The number of non-influenza vaccines administered in children 18 and under has declined by 21.5%, and the percentage of up-to-date statuses is much lower for Medicaid patients[87]. This puts children at risk for vaccine-preventable diseases and their complications[87]. For example, if 90-95% of the population is not vaccinated against the measles, then herd immunity will not be reached and outbreaks of this potentially fatal disease can occur[87]. The CDC posits some strategies to maintain vaccination schedules in the era of COVID and telemedicine[87]:

- Dedicating specific clinics or rooms for sick and well visits.

- Administering vaccinations to patients while they are in their vehicles thus eliminating their need to enter the clinic.

- Closing waiting rooms and having families register on-line.

- Reducing the number of patients on site at any given time.

Should My Child Wear a Mask?

Children under the age of 2 *should not* wear a mask due to risk of suffocation[71].

Children over the age of 2 are recommended to wear a mask. From what I can see in our neighborhood park, this is not happening. Most kids are running around, riding bikes, and *not* socially distancing without a mask. Many adults are mask-less, citing the discomfort and heat of wearing mask as the weather warms. How can we expect our kids to wear them when adults can't stand them? Children are often asymptomatic carriers of the virus, and are thought to be even more infectious than adults given their lack of symptoms and inability to appropriately social distance. Risa grabs her mask of her face whenever I try to get it on. Riaan is much more compliant, as he understands the purpose behind wearing the mask. He even participated in NY Governor Andrew Cuomo's Wear a Mask! PSA contest, where the governor asked New Yorkers to make a 30 second video discussing the importance of wearing a mask. There were some amazing video entries, and I appreciate the governor's efforts to promote mask-wearing and New York pride in a fun way.

Giving Birth During the Pandemic

-Helen Chen, mother of beautiful baby boy Harrison

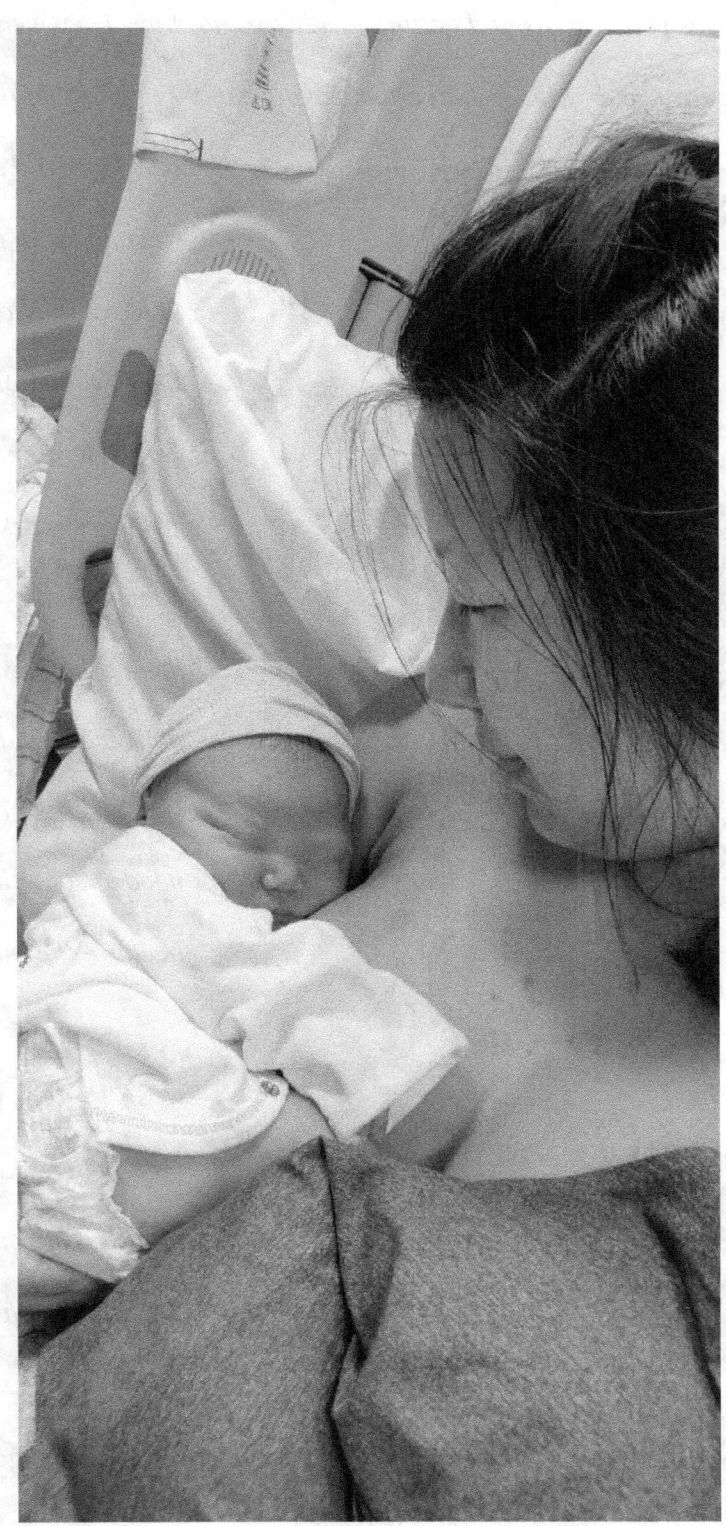

We were nervous, calling the hospital ahead to learn how processes had changed in the pandemic. I was two weeks overdue so I had to get induced. When I arrived at the hospital,

staff checked our temperature. My husband had a temperature of 99 degrees since he was nervous running around getting ready for our stay. They weren't going to let him in due to his temperature, but I also had a temperature of 99 degrees so they permitted him to go with me.

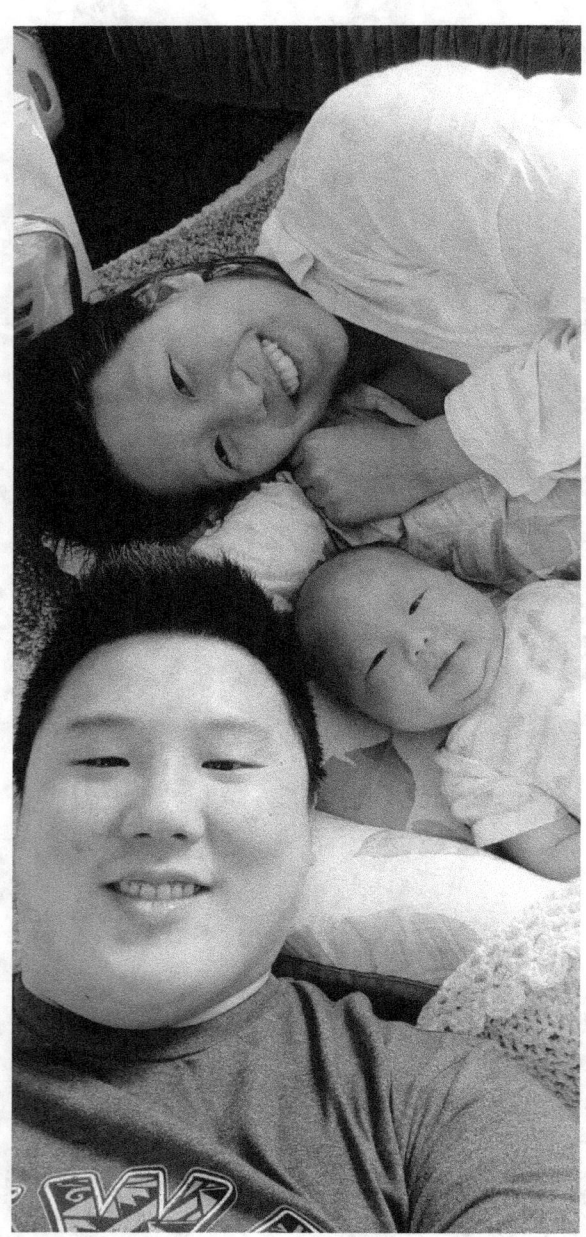

They sprayed down all of our belongings and wrapped it in plastic bags. We weren't allowed to leave the hospital until we were discharged. Luckily the hospital allowed my husband in the delivery room, but only him, no other visitors. We wore masks whenever we had to communicate with the hospital staff, which meant the mask was on the entire time I was delivering and PUSHING. They routinely checked both our temperatures. Whenever we needed someting we would use the call button because the nurse didn't come in often.

Labor was ssoooooo difficult, my body wasn't ready, my tissues were so tight for my baby's big head. I felt like I could barely breathe especially with the mask on, taking that big inhale before pushing was so difficult. The entire bed was soaked with my sweat, and I had a last second episiotomy, I then had post-partum hemorrhage because I was having contractions every 1-3 minutes for the past 14 hours. My uterus was exhausted, I lost over a pint of blood—there were buckets of my blood—I was delusional and not sure what was going on. I wanted to hold my baby but I felt like I could barely move.

We had to be discharged 24 hours after delivery. When we were home, we didn't allow any visitors as a precaution. Even my parents had to see him through a glass door for a month, which was really tough.

The positive is that my husband is working from home! It is great to have him here with us to enjoy the baby in these precious early weeks.

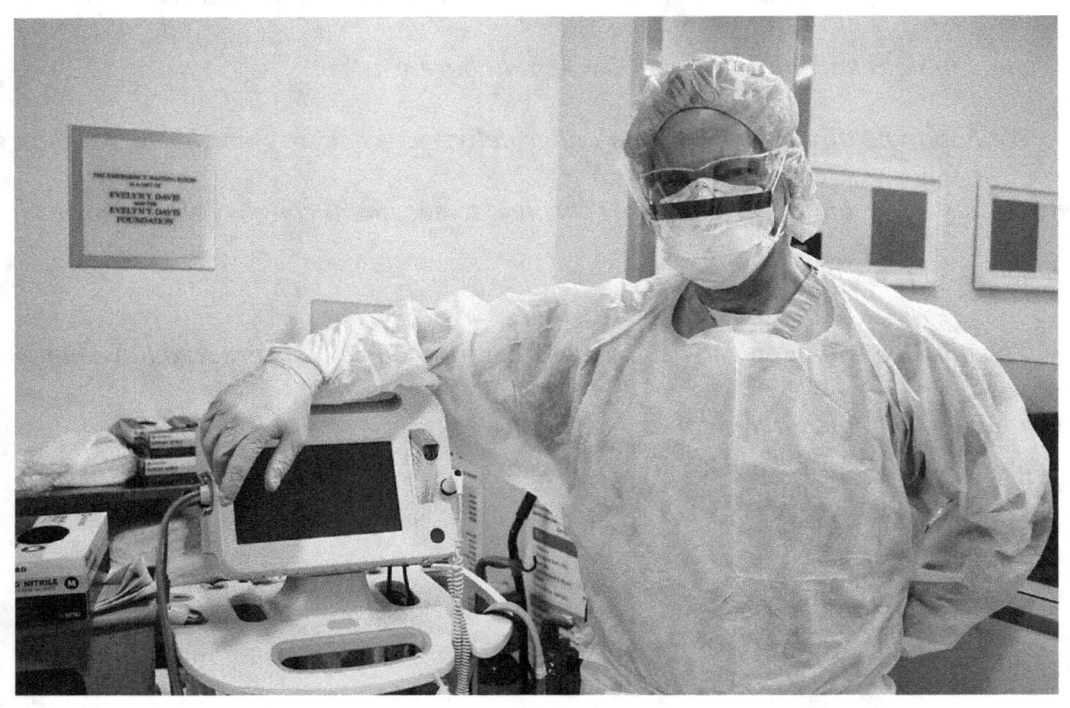

"Do I fear for our patients and each other on the frontlines? Without a doubt. But every life we care for, every life we save, keeps us humble and humane, and full of heart to go on."

-Dr. Michael Stern, MD, Attending Physician, Emergency Department, NYC

Homeschooling while Working from Home

-Aparna Jade, Business Analyst, GA

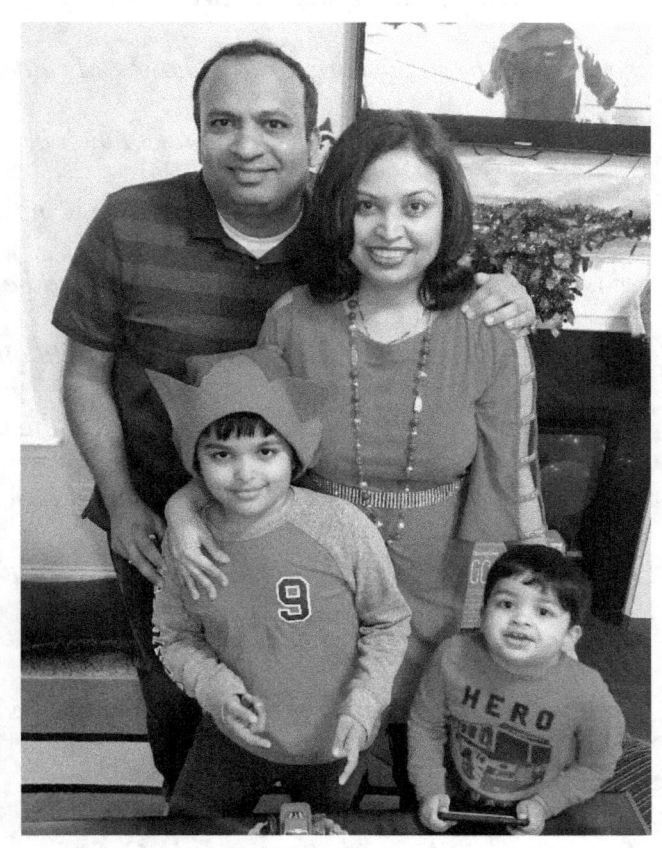

What are some of the challenges you faced homeschooling your children while you and your husband worked from home?
When we went into lockdown, it was sudden. I was at the office and got an email saying that schools were closed. I was still required to work at the office at the time but thankfully my husband was able to work from home. It was very difficult at first. One of my sons is in second grade and the other is 3 years old. For my second grader, he had one hour of Zoom instruction per week and the rest of schooling were packets that we had to do with the children. I didn't like this because if he had any questions then he was unable to speak with the teacher for a week. It was difficult managing both childcare, instruction, and work initially, but we are getting used to the daily routine and are managing better now. Friday mornings are still a challenge since we have both have client meetings at the same time, and we have to rely on TV during these meetings.

Just yesterday I was in a virtual school board meeting. They decided that the next academic year would also start with virtual instruction, but they may change this depending on the infection rate. This is very difficult for working parents. Not many people can afford full-time babysitters. Also, it is difficult for parents of kids with special needs, ADD, or autism to keep them on task all day.

On the positive side, we are able to enjoy being home with each other. My youngest son used to be in daycare for long hours. My elder son always wanted to learn piano and now we finally have the time. We try to take lunch breaks at different times so we can dedicate ourselves to the kids for one hour each. They mostly play together. This month it is very hot outside. My elder son loves to read books, and he reads to the little one. They have bonded a lot in these few months. Before that they would only see each other over the weekends.

Long term, I don't know how being at home will affect their social development. I think the decision to be completely virtual next academic year may change as we pass the peak. The pediatrician on the advisory board recommended that this is not a good time to go back to school. We don't have good data how the virus can be transmitted from one kid to another, but it can be transmitted from child to parent.

Can you describe your experience in Georgia, one of the first states to re-open? *Georgia re-opened early because of the severe economic impact of the lockdown. In our town, there were at least three local businesses that had to shut down permanently. Re-opening was good for businesses, but in terms of the cases it was terrible. We have three hospitals in Columbus that are filled. I used to take my son for bike riding daily at 7pm. An older couple would come out every evening. We would wave to each other and have some small talk. The next day morning the elderly man posted on Facebook that his COVID-19 test came back positive. Despite awaiting a test result, he was still walking outside. Even after his test came back positive he was still going out for a walk. In April and May our neighbors would have pool parties with*

20-25 children in the pool. People are taking this very lightly. This is the reason that the virus is spreading so rapidly.

Masks just became mandatory in Georgia on July 20th. When I go to shops people are not wearing masks. Fortunately, there is one way entry and exit in the shops so people are not facing each other.

In my personal experience, I haven't seen the virus affecting people as severely as you see in the news. In the past 4 or 5 days, our town has not had a new death from the virus. In the news, the virus is portrayed very scarily and so many people are terrified. In April, when I was unloading my groceries into my trunk after shopping, a car stopped near me in the parking lot. There was an old lady in the driver's seat. She said she was 93 years old and was driving around the grocery store parking lot for past 30 minutes. She was looking for someone who could buy groceries for her. I remember her exact words. She said "I am too scared to go inside the shop. I don't wanna die. I need to take care of my husband." Tears rolled out of her eyes while she was talking. She had a list of groceries and money in her hand. I told her I could absolutely help her. I shopped for her and loaded her groceries into her car. I gave her my number to call if she needs help in future.

CHAPTER 13: COVID-19 IN NEW YORK

"They showed up. God Bless them."

-Andrew Cuomo, Governor of New York, on the heroic response of essential workers

In the early days of the pandemic when schools were closed and businesses shut, I would look outside my apartment window and see Seton Park bustling with activity—it seemed more so than ever now that parents and their children were homebound. It took a while for people to realize the seriousness of the disease or to feel personal impact that motivated them to stay home. But as cases rose exponentially and the government started enforcing social isolation procedures, the scene soon changed.

New York City was hardest hit by the virus, with more than 18,000 confirmed and 5,000 4,000 probable COVID-19 related deaths[136]. Almost half the infections in the country are in the city that never sleeps[98], leaving streets barren and unrecognizable. City sounds have been replaced with the wail of sirens, and it is no wonder one of my daughter's first words is "ambulance."

From March 11th through April 27th more than 27,000 NYC residents have died, which is six times the normal city death count during this season[90]. This suggests that either some

COVID-19 deaths are unaccounted for or New Yorkers are dying at increased rates of other illnesses during the pandemic as well, possibly as a result of decreased medical care for non-COVID related conditions.

No event in recent history has claimed as many New Yorker lives. The most recent cause of mass casualty in the city were the terror attacks of the World Trade Centers on September 11th, which resulted in a fraction of the deaths caused by the COVID-19 pandemic.

Testing

The state has tested over 2.2 million individuals as of June 3rd, and is averaging 50,000 tests per day[8]. The current positivity rate in NY is 1.7%, but continues to approach 5% in NYC in early June[114]. Testing is prioritized for patients at risk for the disease and those who are symptomatic, though anyone is able to obtain a test at this time.

Economic Impact

Over the first 5 weeks of the pandemic, 1.2 million New York residents filed unemployment claims[99]. As the social net has expanded and tax revenue lost, NYC is experiencing its most severe economic recession since the Great Depression. As a result, significant budget cuts are expected. Margaret Besheer of VOA quotes Governor Andrew Cuomo, "We are at a point financially where we have a $10- $15 billion deficit. We have real financial problems right now." Governor Cuomo has issued an Americans First Law stating that a corporation cannot receive government funding if it does not rehire the same number of workers it had prior to the pandemic.

Assisting the Community

Throughout the pandemic, three free meals were provided to any NYC residents at multiple sites throughout the city. Meals could be delivered straight to the doors of our vulnerable elderly population. Housing was provided to homeless and essential workers who did not want to risk infecting their families. In order to prevent people from becoming homeless, NY state suspended all evictions for those experiencing a financial hardship due to COVID-19 until August 20th, 2020[42].

Library System

The closure that most affected my family was that of the public library system. The library is my family's second home. The librarians have known my children since they were born (I started reading to them when they were in the womb!). My son developed his love of reading at the library, my daughter took her first steps at the library, and for me the library has always been a refuge of comfort, friendship, and knowledge. NY closed its public library system on March 14th, and has plans to reopen some branches in July. Millions of people rely on the library every day—for books, computer access, socialization, and study space. The library provides infinite and universal access to knowledge and, while necessary to prevent social interaction, its closure is a blow to learning and development across the nation. The New York Public Library (NYPL) system has tried to remain engaged with the community by providing e-books and daily homework help to students. The library encouraged families to keep borrowed materials with all fines frozen during the pandemic.

Metropolitan Transportation Authority (MTA)

Throughout the pandemic, the MTA continued to operate in order to transport essential workers to and from work. Subway service was suspended between 1am and 5am for deep cleaning of the trains. They are utilizing over 150 ultraviolet light machines to treat the trains, with plans to obtain more. NY has dispensed over 1 million masks and 500,000 bottles of hand sanitizers to MTA workers[110]. Families of MTA workers who died from COVID-19 are being compensated by the state government to honor the loss of their loved ones, who sacrificed their lives to keep others safe.

Re-opening New York

As of June 8th, Long Island and Mid-Hudson Valley have met all 7 criteria necessary for phase 1 re-opening. NYC entered phase 1 on June 8th. As of June 10th, the Mid-Hudson Valley, Long Island, Capital Region, Western and Central NY, Finger Lakes, Mohawk Valley, North Country, and Southern Tier have all been permitted to begin phase 2[110].

In phase 2 of re-opening, outdoor dining at restaurants will be permitted and places of worship may open at 25% of capacity.[110] Hair salons and office spaces will be opened. As NY reopens, there will still be significant changes in place. Facilities will be sanitized more often. Social distancing will remain in place. Diners and workers will be seated six feet apart (though up to 10 people per restaurant table are permitted). Diners and staff will be required to wear masks[109].

Throughout the reopening process, the state government has a plan to monitor progress and spikes of cases, with plans of contact tracing when necessary.

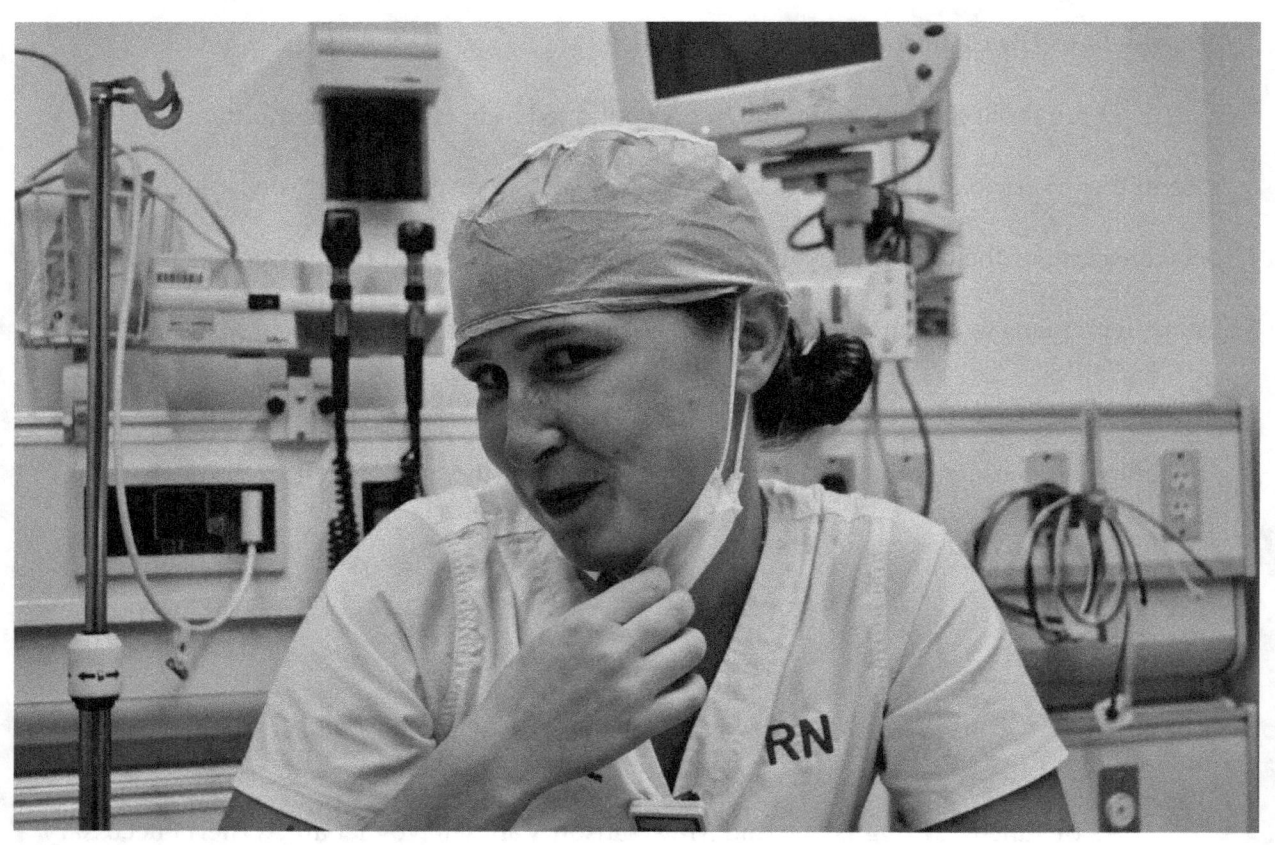

"Being a nurse through this unprecedented time has been humbling, heartbreaking, and beautiful in some surprising little ways. You really start to realize that the most important thing is just the people. To be with them, to savor them, and to love them, especially when life feels super big and scary. Isolation has a way of telling us that of all things, we need each other the most."

- **Adelene Egan, Registered Nurse, Emergency Department, NYC**

Letter from Dr. Michael Prodromou, MD, Pulmonary Critical Care/ICU Attending Redeployed to Mt. Sinai Queens, NYC

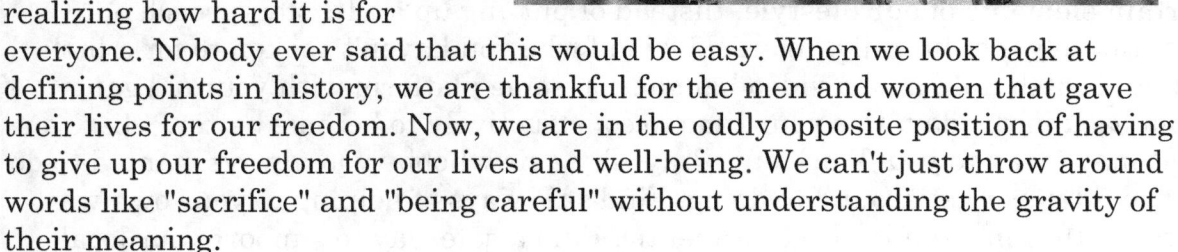

March 24th:

To my dear friends and family,

A few days into this and I am realizing how hard it is for everyone. Nobody ever said that this would be easy. When we look back at defining points in history, we are thankful for the men and women that gave their lives for our freedom. Now, we are in the oddly opposite position of having to give up our freedom for our lives and well-being. We can't just throw around words like "sacrifice" and "being careful" without understanding the gravity of their meaning.

If you read or watch the news, you will hear about all the things that the medical community, private companies, and the government are doing to help fix this. THEY are working on a vaccine. THEY are working on a cure. THEY are making more masks. THEY are bringing a floating hospital to New York.

I think that we should stop relying solely on THEM, and acknowledge how important YOUR contributions are, too. Realize that YOU are a hero too. YOU are making a sacrifice, and YOU are suffering emotionally, socially, economically, and physically just like everybody else. Yes, our doctors, nurses, pharmacists, and service people are all facing a more obvious threat every day they go to work - but do not discount YOUR sacrifice, and YOUR contribution to the cause. By letting go of much of your life that was taken for granted just weeks ago, and staying home, YOU are helping decrease the spread of this disease. Do not feel helpless - you are all doing your part. It is easy to live in panic and feel helpless by all we hear and see during these unprecedented times - but don't give in - the power is in YOUR hands (so long as you wash them for 20 seconds!!).

By quarantining yourself from loved ones because you may have been exposed, you are making a sacrifice that can save lives. By leaving your familiar and comfortable set up to go to a safer place, you are making a sacrifice that can save lives. Know that you are making a difference - but also realize that you are not alone. You may be confined to the same limited space, interacting physically with the same few people, but you are NOT alone. We all share the same concerns, fears, doubts, confusion and inconveniences. We are all in this together.

I realize I have been living in my own bubble for the past few years. How did I start living such a fast-paced lifestyle, where the majority of my human interaction became a never-ending barrage of texts, memes or Facebook/Instagram (IG) stories? In the past few days I have been able to reconnect to voices from different times of my life - friends from high school, college, medical school, residency, fellowship. After a few 15 minute conversations with friends that I had not spoken to in months, I realized how much the way we live our life can interfere with and depersonalize our friendships.

I can't help but think that a portion of our discomfort stems from the detox of certain elements of our lifestyle. Instead of putting up an IG story, reach out (figuratively, not literally) to an old friend who you haven't spoken to for a little bit, and catch up! Make a video hangout on some platform with your old gang from back in the day. Use your time to constructively to become better, whatever that may mean to you. Work out. Pray. Try a new hobby you always wanted to do but could never get around to doing. Find safe ways of helping in your own way, because that in itself is also therapeutic. Find a safe way to support your local businesses, while keeping that curve flat.

We must stay united and steadfast in our resolve. It won't be easy. Stay positive, and when you feel overwhelmed, phone a friend - chances are they won't be busy and they'll happy to hear from you. Don't let the politics make you lose sight of what really matters, and don't worry, everybody with an opinion will have plenty of time to point their sterile fingers at each other later on. If you are worried about finances, you are not alone. Let's beat this and rebuild.

You are strong. Thank you for ALL for your contributions. Through our collective efforts, sacrifice and care, we will get through this.

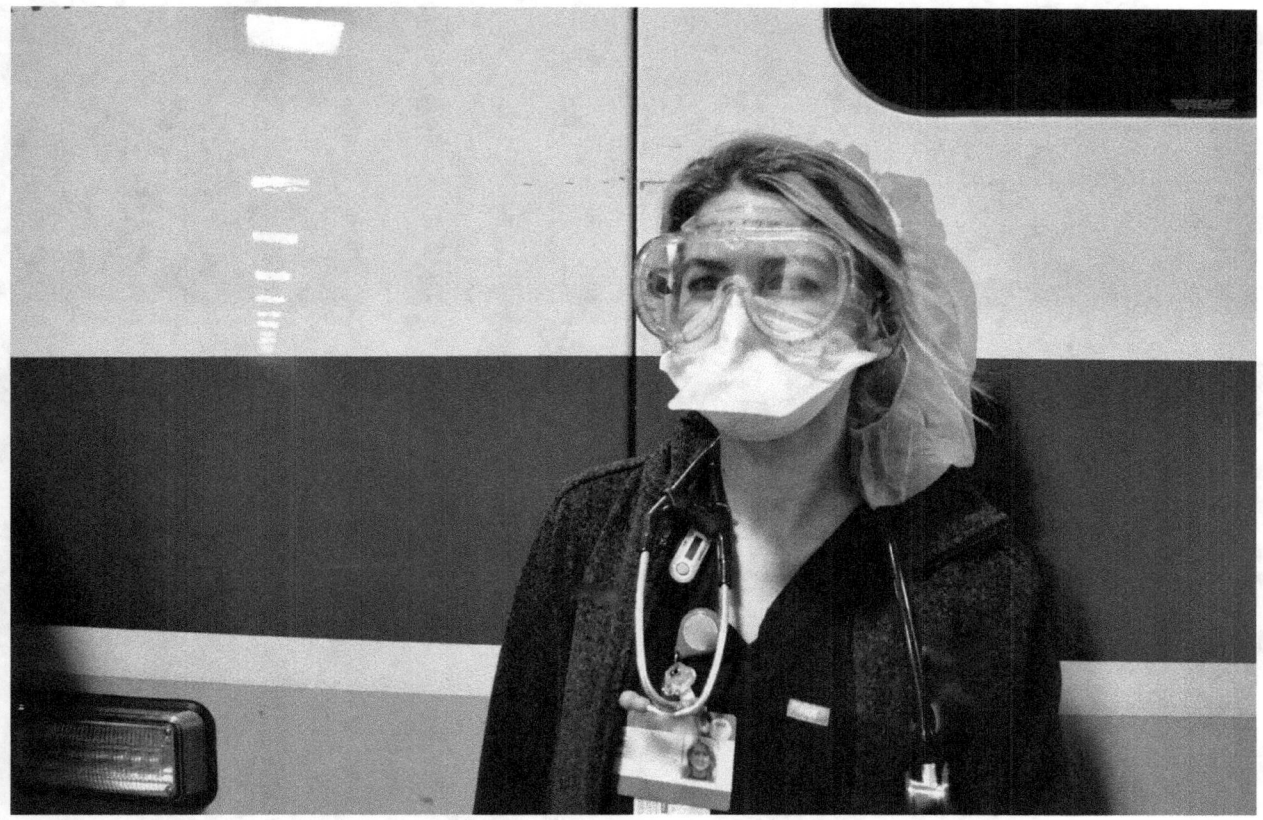

"We saved lives before and will keep saving lives now. There is no virus more vigorous than us."

-Ashley Green, Physician Assistant, Emergency Department, NYC

CHAPTER 14:

COVID-19 IN NURSING HOMES

"Given their congregate nature and resident population served (e.g., older adults often with underlying chronic medical conditions), nursing home populations are at high risk of being affected by respiratory pathogens like COVID-19."

-Centers for Disease Control and Prevention (CDC)

In the early days of the pandemic, nursing homes were requiring patients to be COVID negative before we could discharge our patients to them. This was a challenge even for our asymptomatic patients, as we could often not obtain infectious diseases approval for the swab when the patient did not medically require it. As we approached the peak and beds were rapidly being converted into ICU space, it would have been impossible to keep medical stable patients in house. In her interview with me, Dr. Gina Kang, a geriatrician at Yale New Haven Hospital, discusses the challenges she faced discharging patients from Yale to nursing homes given that many CT nursing homes did not accept any patients. Although hit hard, Yale was not as severely hit as New York and she was able to keep medically stable patients on their unit for 1 or 2 weeks while family members selected facilities or prepared for home discharge.

On March 25th, Governor Cuomo mandated that nursing homes accept COVID-19 patients from hospitals in order to provide placement for medically stable patients who were unsafe to return home. At that time, CDC guidelines recommended that nursing homes have a specific place to quarantine nursing home patients before they could accept COVID-19 positive patients.

Nursing homes have since been brutally affected by COVID-19 given their high population of elderly patients with multiple comorbidities. As of June 21st, there have been 51,000 nursing home deaths, accounting for nearly 40% of COVID-related deaths across the country. As of early July, there have been 6,200 deaths of nursing home patients in New York State[52]. It is likely that this is an underrepresentation, as NY only tallies patients who died in a nursing facility, excluding those who contracted the virus in a nursing facility and went on to die in a hospital. Nevertheless, it still represents more than 1/10 of COVID related nursing home deaths nationwide and is higher than Florida, which has many more nursing home residents than New York. Governor Cuomo has been criticized for the high death rate of nursing home patients. Critics say that the most vulnerable members of the population should have been protected during the pandemic, and nursing home residents are at the front of this list. On the other hand, where were these patients to go? Even without COVID-19, we often have a difficult time discharging patients who are unsafe to go home to the most appropriate facilities. Insurances deny coverage, family members are resistant to send their loved ones to facilities with less than desirable care and conditions, and facilities often have strict criteria regarding whom they can accept (many don't take patients on dialysis, ventilators, with tracheostomies or PEG tubes, or those who require bariatric beds). There are several possible reasons for the higher death rate in New York: it may not have been feasible for many crowded NY nursing homes to separate COVID positive and negative patients; a lack of PPE early in the crisis could have facilitated spread between patients and asymptomatic healthcare workers; the warmer temperature in Florida may have limited the contagiousness of the virus; and NY experienced peak COVID cases earlier than other states, many of which are experiencing rising cases now in mid-June as NY cases decrease.

One possible solution to this problem could have been to discharge nursing home patients to a COVID-only space—either a nursing home dedicated to COVID patients or a field hospital, the Comfort ship, or the Javitz center—any designated space for medically stable COVID patients who were unsafe for discharge home. There is no easy answer, but as Dr. Katie Rief says, the important thing is reversing course when we realize our mistakes.

Given the high rate of COVID-19 fatalities in nursing home residents, in May Governor Cuomo issued an executive order that prohibited hospitals from discharging COVID positive patients to nursing homes. It also required that all skilled nursing facilities test their employees twice per week, COVID-19 positive patients be kept on separate floors from those without the virus, and that all positive cases and fatalities be reported to families within 24 hours. By this time the number of COVID cases was declining and there was more time to formulate appropriate discharge plans for patients, both COVID positive and negative.

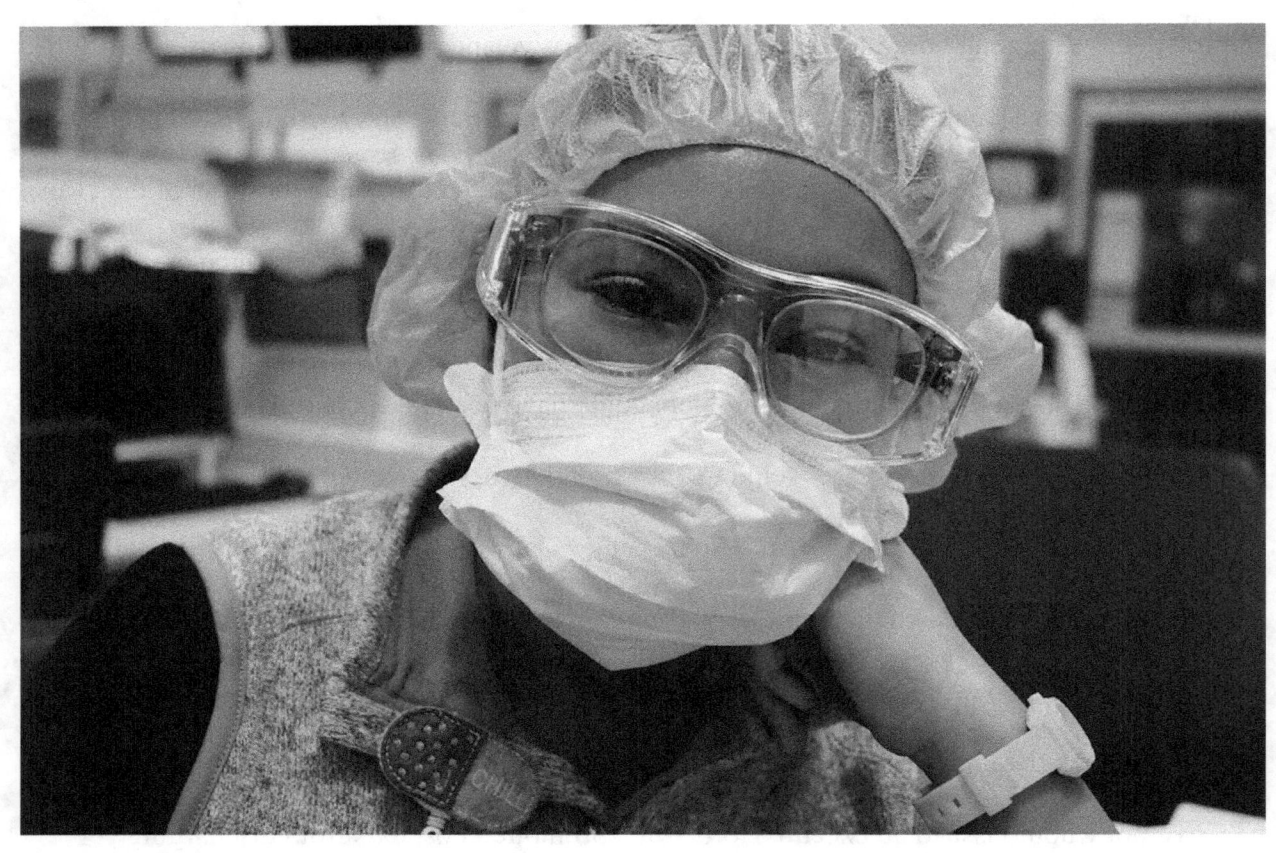

"Being on the frontlines during the COVID-19 pandemic serves as a reminder that we may all come from different walks of life, but at the end of the day our humanity binds us together."

-Delis Cedeno, Technician, Emergency Department, NYC

Caring for COVID patients in Multiple Settings

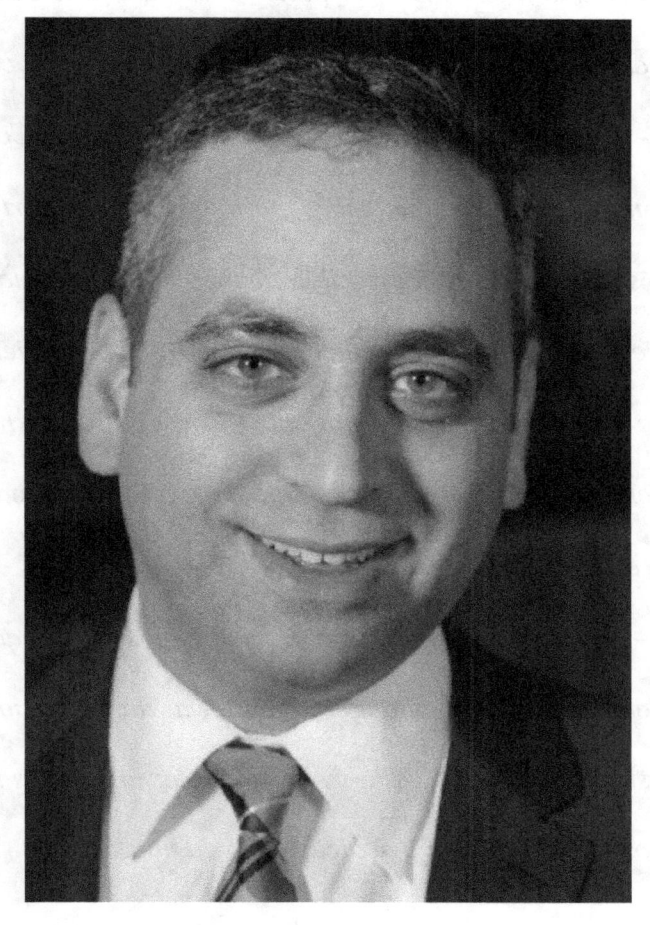

—*Dr. Samuel Rosenberg, DO, Attending Physician, NYC*

You work in many settings—inpatient, outpatient, as a consultant, and as medical director of a subacute rehabilitation facility. What was it like to work in each of these settings during the pandemic? *As the reality of the coronavirus set in, the rehab medicine team was affected on all fronts.*

1- Outpatient: Our outpatient operations were shut completely, with exception made for emergencies (such as baclofen pump refills, severe pain requiring injection). Most of our doctors transitioned to seeing patients via Telehealth visits. This was not done prior to the crisis, so our doctors, staff, and patients had to learn to negotiate the technology and perform these visits successfully.

2 - Inpatient: Initially our unit was closed to Covid patients. In early April as the first of the hospitalized Covid patients were stabilized, we created protocols to assess and admit these patients. While initially these patients were the minority on our unit, the situation rapidly evolved to where most our patients now are post-Covid patients. The demand continued to increase and we established 2 additional units to focus on these patients.

3 - Consults: One of the crises that occurred with Covid-19 was the shortage of PPE. Our consults were screened more thoroughly as an effort to conserve PPE (so we weren't going in to see patients unnecessarily), furthermore we would not have the resident and the attending see patients together; rather one would see the patient and then discuss afterwards. In May, we started seeing many more post-Covid patients who had complicated clinical courses and were ready for rehab. This led to a significant increase in consultation requests and the need to establish more bed capacity.

4 – Subacute Rehabilitation: Early in the crisis I made the decision to avoid consulting in the Hebrew Home. My thought process was that I did not want to act as a vector between the two institutions. I was available by phone for any issues they needed assistance with. The Hebrew Home did establish a dedicated Covid unit.

What percentage of your inpatients have COVID-19? *In April the percentage was low, but has been steadily increasing through May. As of today, June 3rd, 60% of the patients on my service are post-Covid.*

How did COVID-19 change rehab in the unit? *Once it became apparent that Covid patients would be admitted, we had to establish guidelines for which patients would be kept on isolation and which could have restrictions lifted. In order for isolation restrictions to be lifted, patients had to be asymptomatic and have two negative Covid swabs greater than 24* hours apart. Patients in isolation had therapy in their rooms only. As with the rest of the hospital, any staff entering the Covid patient rooms had to follow the hospital guidelines for PPE.

How was the camaraderie among your team? *The staff on the unit had excellent camaraderie throughout this crisis. There was and is a strong sense of team and the need to serve these patients.*

Were staff infected? *We had 3 staff members who were infected. None of them severely.*

Can you describe some of the patient experiences that most affected you/are most memorable to you? *I felt very sad for these patients. Due to the crisis, none of them were allowed to have visitors. Additionally, staff typically avoided these rooms and only went in when needed. When they did go in they were dressed completely in PPE (hair covering, 2 masks, face shield, and gown). These patients were essentially cut off from their loved ones and allowed limited social interaction, and when they did have interactions the people were completely covered up. This meant these patients had not seen loved ones and people looking normal for weeks.*

Have you seen any treatments that helped? *A few of the treatments that appeared to be very helpful anecdotally were proning and convalescent serum. Some patients reported to me that they felt much better and their course really improved after the convalescent serum treatments.*

What would you like people to know about COVID-19? *The disease can be devastating. I have seen patients in their 30s and 40s with no prior health issues who were severely affected and remain with long term medical issues as a result of the disease. It is important to remain vigilant as restrictions ease, especially if they have had exposure to anyone sick with the virus.*

CHAPTER 15: HOSPITAL RESPONSE TO THE NOVEL CORONAVIRUS

"May God guide and watch over all of us who are in the frontlines during this time of crisis. I am praying for the patients and families whose loved ones are in our care."

-Sonieta Reyes, Registered Nurse, Emergency Department, NYC

I look down at the empty streets of New York, normally bustling with energy. Where have all the people gone? Surely patients still need care and healthcare providers are still coming to work? Yet even by the hospital, probably the busiest place in the pandemic, the streets are devoid of life.

Infection Control

At the three facilities at which I worked during the pandemic, there has always the appropriate PPE that I needed, including surgical masks, N95 masks, gowns, and gloves. I attribute this to the foresight of the administrations in securing PPE and the resourcefulness of their staff in using their resources carefully. Media suggests this is not the case throughout the country, and fears over PPE shortage have been expressed in several of the accounts you read in this book. In Missouri, one family filed a death claim on behalf of a 69-year-old nurse who died from COVID-19, stating that she was not provided appropriate PPE from her facility. When discussing her husband's death in this book, Priya Jose told me that neither she nor her husband had access to appropriate PPE while they worked in a New York hospital.

Limitation of Patient Visitors

Patient's family members are an essential part of their medical care. If you have been a patient yourself, you know how much the support of your loved one means to you when you are in your sickest, most vulnerable state. During my two pregnancies, I loved having my husband in the labor & delivery room with me, to care for me, talk to, and revel in the precious and exhausting moments of delivering our children. And I am a fully functional, strong woman. I see patients who are blind from stroke, unable to communicate but for the blinking of their eyes due to locked-in-syndrome, or unable to get out of bed on their own because of recent amputations. Caregivers are such an important part of these patients' recoveries, both for emotional and physical support. In our TBI unit, patients are already at a high rate of depression, but mental illness has soared since they have been kept isolated from their family members but for phone and video chat. Worse, patients who succumbed to the virus in the hospital did not have the comfort of their families at their sides.

The Rise of Telemedicine

As resources shifted to hospitalized COVID-19 patients and non-urgent surgeries and outpatient visits were postponed, many providers looked to telemedicine to continue to care for patients and to keep their practices afloat. I have been interested in the prospect of telemedicine for years, as it is often inconvenient and physically challenging for patients to visit their doctors, not to mention expensive when considering commute and NYC parking rates. Telemedicine can be a practical and accessible treatment mode for many patient encounters. Prior to the pandemic, it appeared to me that one of the main reasons for its infrequent utilization was lack of reimbursement for such visits by insurance companies. As of this writing in May, almost all outpatient visits at the three hospitals where I worked were through telemedicine, with only emergent visits seen in-person. In May, I did several telemedicine visits for spinal cord injury patients. According to one physician, limitations of telemedicine include inability to perform direct physical examination, occasionally poor-quality video, and technical difficulties at the patient end that are often challenging. He states that though not ideal, under the circumstances, telemedicine is the best tool we have to check on our outpatients, address minor issues, assist in triaging patients, and provide educations and guidance.

Dr. Niurka Visconti, a primary care physician in Connecticut, says her practice closed in March and she has conducted primarily telemedicine visits since then. "We are a 40-year-old practice and have a lot of patients who still need care—our service has been overwhelmed with phone calls since our practice closed. Telemedicine has been useful so we can see patients who still really need care. It is easier, but not optimal since I cannot physically examine my patients. It's something I would only use in an emergency like this."

Burnout

Prior to the pandemic, levels of burnout and mental distress among healthcare workers soared. During my residency, there was always an emphasis on preventing burnout and promoting wellbeing. In the time of COVID-19, levels of burnout and utter exhaustion have escalated among healthcare providers. Seeing constant death, and filling the role of family at dying patients' bedsides has taken its toll. Such harrowing scenes can be traumatic even for the well-trained health care provider, who is accustomed to treating very sick patients on a daily basis.

On top of psychological stress, healthcare workers are facing the physical stresses of contracting the virus. As of mid-July, 782 healthcare workers across the United States have succumbed to the virus[135]. In the wise words of New Jersey nurse practitioner Joanne Sherstein, "all the applause in the world can never make up for their loss."

Letter from Dr. Michael Prodromou, MD, Pulmonary Critical Care/ICU Attending Redeployed to Mt. Sinai Queens, NYC

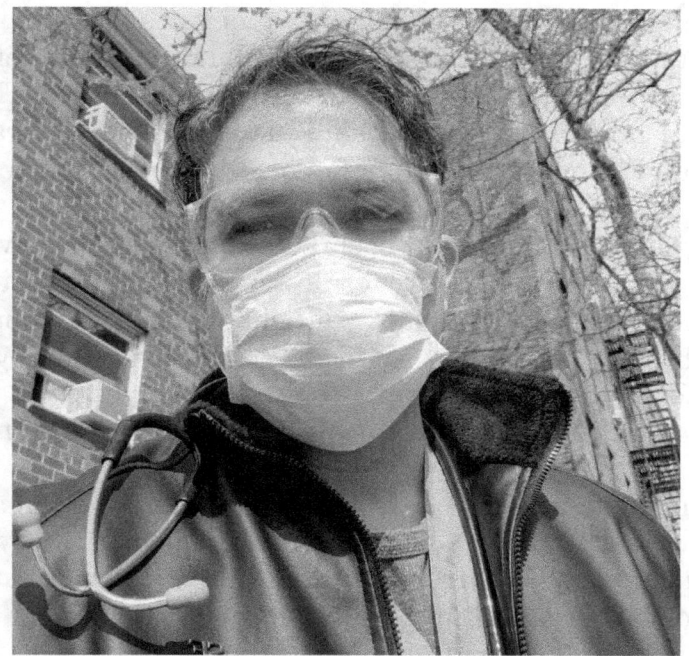

April 7th:

To my dear family and friends,

I hope you are doing well. Quarantine is taking a physical, mental, and emotional toll on us. I have been dealing with separation from my loved ones, sadness over the loss of a colleague, fear of friends and family contracting the disease, and concern for my own health while on the frontlines. The news features depressing statistics, freak stories about unexpected deaths, and political finger pointing. Even a random cough is enough to get my mind racing.

Though I am sure we share many such emotions, it doesn't mean we must feel defeated and helpless. We must maintain a healthy balance of hope, awareness of the facts, and responsible action. Stay informed, know the dangers, act intelligently. But also deflect from the negative news and hysteria. Give your mind a moment of peace!

Quarantine life has shown me that we are so lucky to live such privileged lifestyles. We had basic freedoms that we took for granted – and by that I don't mean political freedoms, but social freedoms, such as being able to travel anywhere we wanted, freedom to eat communally, freedom to give a hug without concern for disease transmission. Freedom should never be taken for granted.

Now a new enemy has challenged our way of life and life itself. This is a fight we are ALL in together – everyone has suffered and everybody has an important role in the battle.

History will look at this moment as one of the greatest challenges of the century. We will speak to future generations of how the world turned upside down in a matter of weeks, and together we did our part to defeat the virus and return to normalcy. We were challenged emotionally, physically, financially, and found the strength to recover - strength we never knew we had. We will tell our youth about wiping down groceries, suspending life indefinitely, wearing masks everywhere we went, and hoarding toilet paper. These times will forever be part of our fabric, and we will share stories about quarantine life, the sacrifices that we had to make, and the memories of those who are gone but never forgotten.

This letter is not about social distancing because we have been talking about that for what seems like forever now - if you aren't social distancing by now, you are either living under a rock, selfish, or a fool. My hope today is to remind you that within our world that seems to be riddled with negative emotions, physical suffering and chaos, there are still some positives. In order to appreciate them, you have to keep the right mindset, perspective and attitude.

Give your mind and body the break it needs from all the negative news to keep a positive attitude. Do not discount the power that you wield by social distancing and denying this virus the fuel it needs to spread. Realize that your efforts and sacrifices are working!

Personally, I want to thank you for all your support at the beginning of my redeployment – I was dreading going to work, and all your words of encouragement, in the form of texts, calls, or Facebook messages made a world of a difference. Thank you!

In these past few days, I have seen the human condition at its worst, but humanity at its finest. I'm so proud of how we banded together to combat this virus. You should be proud of your efforts too. Stay strong and safe everybody! There is light at the end of the tunnel.

Six degrees apart, six degrees together

-Ansel Oommen, Clinical Lab Technologist, NYC

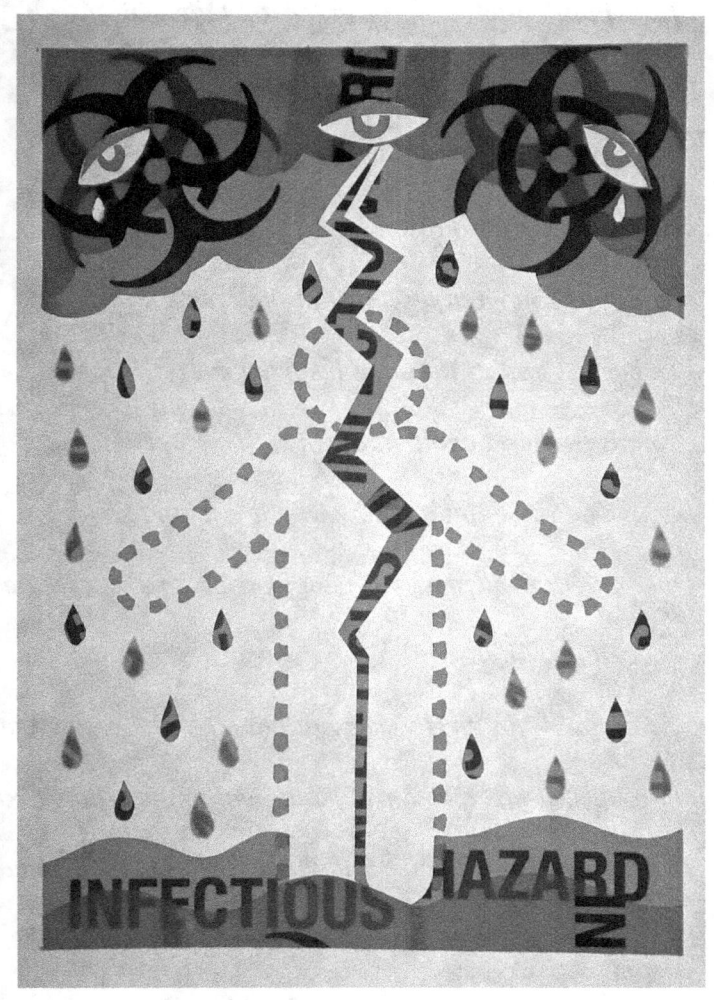

What was it like to work in the lab during the pandemic? *We were the first hospital in New York to have a positive case. Our department was monitoring the situation carefully even before this case was admitted. Typically, four of my colleagues and I work the night shift and we are a really close team. The pandemic split us up. The department asked for volunteers to test COVID samples. A lot of people did not want to volunteer because they were elderly or had a preexisting condition. There were people with kids who were afraid to transmit it to their families. Even if you did volunteer, you had to pass a competency to be able to conduct the test. I was the only one who met all these criteria.*

Does this mean you were the only one processing lab tests at night during the peak of the pandemic? *Yes, for at least 20 days in the beginning I was the only one, and I was working all my days off because there was no one else who could process the tests. I cannot explain to you what an unusual time period this has been. I got all the samples from every NYP campus—when I came into work, there were buckets of tests. And the phone is ringing off the hook. Doctors want to know why it's taking so long to get the test results for their patients. One patient needs an emergency procedure and we need to know the test result before proceeding. And I can't even answer the phone because then I can't process the results.*

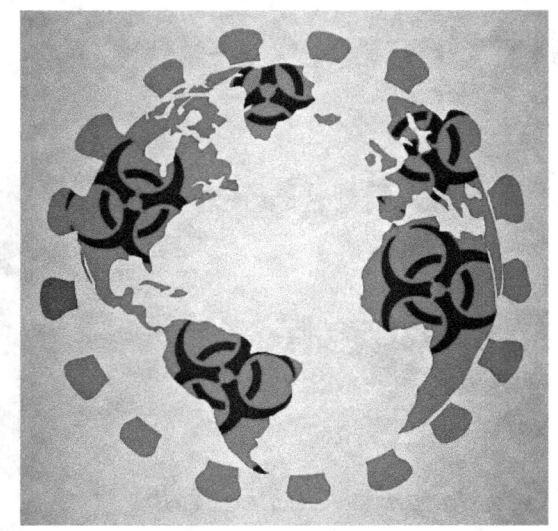

I was the first to see patient's results. I saw the high positivity rate before the clinicians. It has a real psychological impact. Some cases are positive, some are negative, some are indeterminate. But what does that really mean? In these cases, I worked closely with the director to determine what the next step should be. There are two main gene sequences we look at with the PCR nasal swab. What if a patient is positive in one sequence and not the other? What is the significance of this?

Furthermore, I was alone. Before the pandemic, my four colleagues and I were together in the same room all day. Now I was physically isolated, processing tests by myself all night. Every day I went to see them for about 10 minutes, to check-in and see how they were doing. My director Dr. Green would stay in the lab for several days straight to help process specimens. This is not typical and I was so appreciative. Eventually other techs also passed the competency and many worked double shifts to help me. It was really touching.

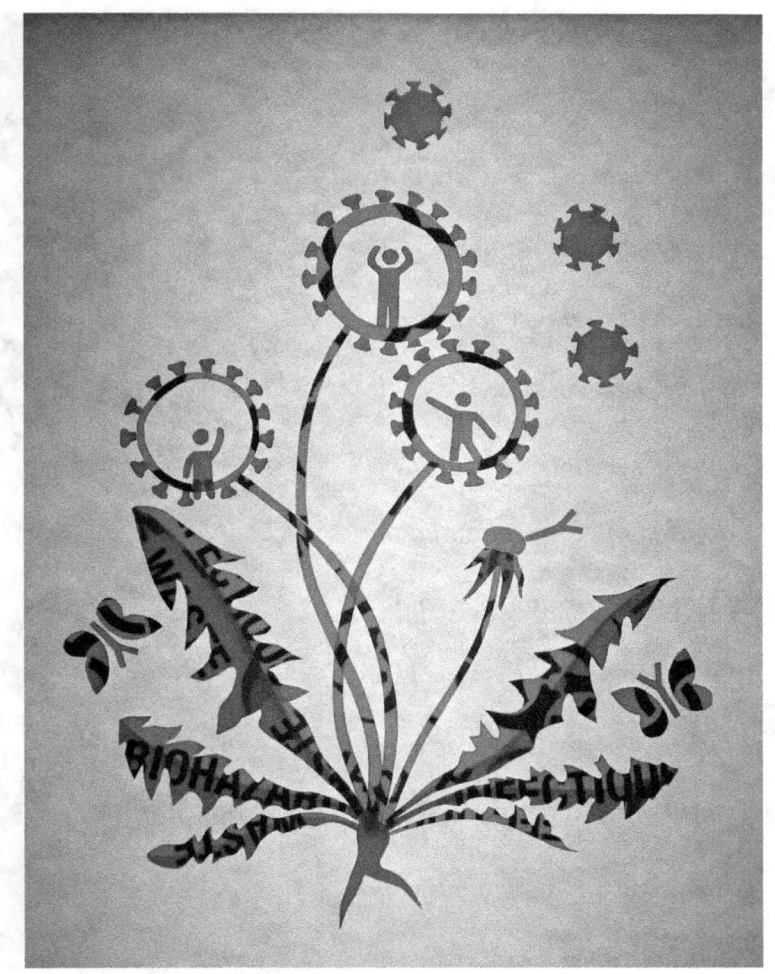

Did you fear exposure while you processed the samples? *Our department exercised caution and all samples were sent in a clear bag. If anything was leaking, we would cancel the specimen. Everything was bleached before and after testing. I didn't feel at risk from working in the lab. I was more scared of community transmission.*

You were studying grief and family counseling prior to the pandemic. How did this training impact you during the pandemic? *I remember one instance in the very beginning—my colleague and I were working together on slides and she suddenly asked me, "What will* *happen to my kids if I die?" It was so unexpected. I think she is in her late 30s. The mental health professional in me felt we needed to pause to talk and address her feelings. We stopped looking at slides. I said I don't know and validated the fact that this is an uncertain time for all of us. Even working as techs, we are a source of emotional support for our colleagues and communities. The lab is a lot more dynamic than people think. In this crisis,*

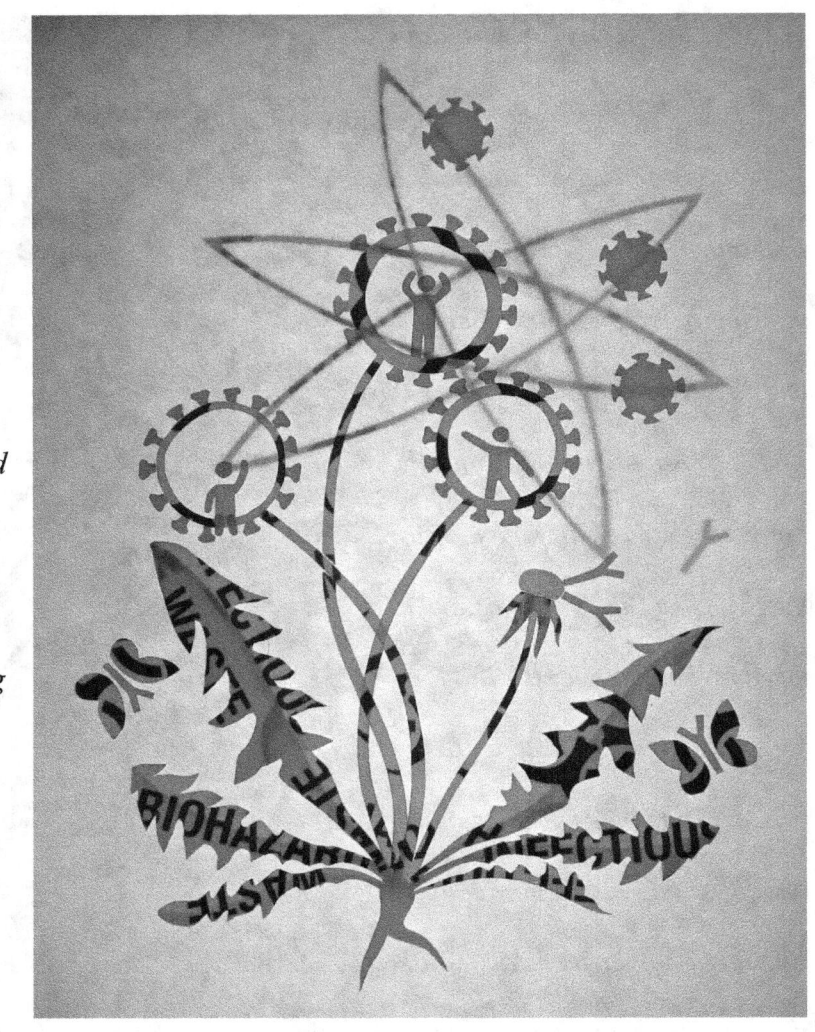

the ED ad ICU receive the adulation—and they deserve it. Their world is as foreign to me as mine is to theirs. People often don't realize that those who work in the lab see patients too. Not in the conventional sense, but we see their stories. I see the same patients multiple times a day when I process their labs and can understand how their conditions progress. This week I kept seeing the samples of a child until I saw a post-mortem sample. I knew the child died and I felt deep sadness, even though I had never met them. It's hard to explain that grief to other healthcare professionals.

How do you think New York handled the pandemic? *New York hospitals led by example. Not every state responded the way we would expect. New Yorkers rallied together. You don't see us rioting. I think that speaks to how tough we are. There is a coolness to New Yorkers that came through during this pandemic.*

You made some beautiful artwork related to the pandemic. Can you tell us about this?

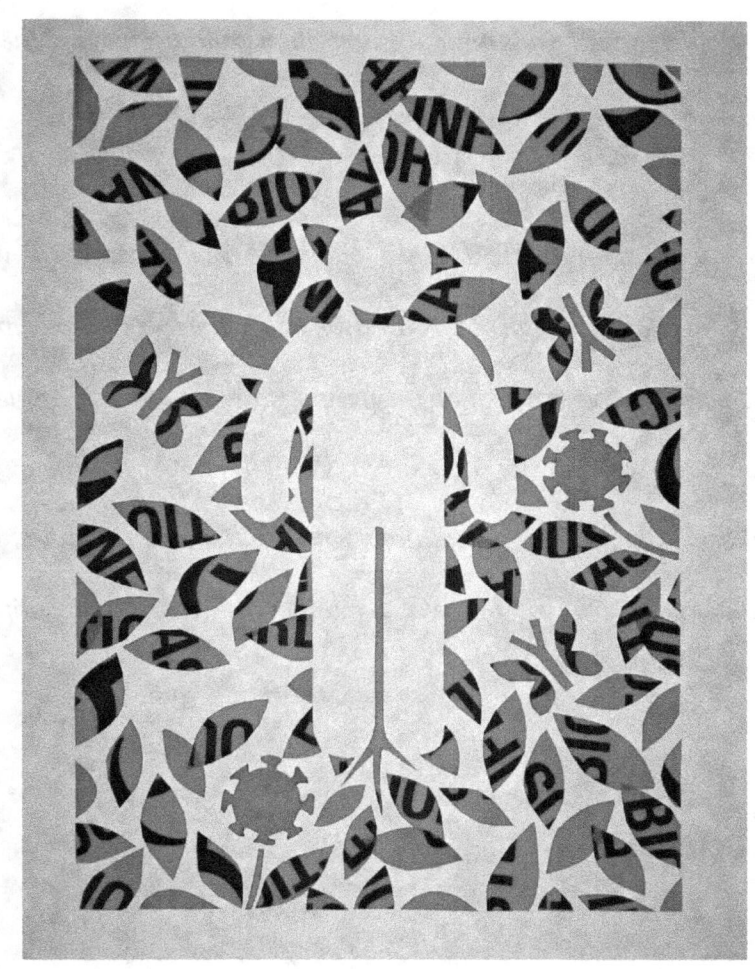

When I was working 20 nights in a row I felt physical and psychological fatigue. My first degree is in toxicology and I see art as a way of metabolizing your frustrations. Greif and loss- they're emotions that need to be processed, and if you let them fester, they can envelop you. In this case, I used biohazard labels in my artwork.

A lot of animals use color to alert people that they are dangerous. The purpose of the biohazard label is to alert people to danger. You want people to be focused when you're handling the material. Orange and black are not part of my color palette but it felt right in this case. My first piece was inspired by the cytokine storm, one of the most dangerous aspects of this disease, which makes me think of someone being struck by a bolt of lightning.

April 22nd is Earth day. After my shift, I walked down the street. You hear the birds singing, see the flowers blooming, but there are so few people in the street that it feels like "silent spring." I thought of Rachel Carson, who wrote the book to alert people of how pesticides were killing animals and plants and destroying the environment. In this case we have Silent Spring because the streets are devoid of life.

"Six degrees apart, six degrees together:" The coronavirus virion is unusual because it has these bulbous spike proteins all over its surface. It reminds me of a dandelion seed head. They are considered weeds since they are easily spread and people don't like them. This piece is meant to show how COVID spreads and to convey resiliency. A dandelion can grow in the concrete and in harsh conditions where other plants cannot. We have to adapt in the pandemic to grow and thrive. Even though we are six feet apart, we are still together.

CHAPTER 16: COVID-19 IN AMERICA

"WE WILL WIN THIS WAR." When we achieve this victory, we will emerge stronger and more united than ever before!"

-President Donald J. Trump

The first reported case of COVID-19 in America occurred in Iowa on January 24th in a woman in her 60s who had returned from travel in Wuhan, China. Her husband was found to be positive thereafter, and by the end of the month, cases were being reported in Washington State. On March 13th, the United Stated declared a state of emergency[87]. Since then COVID-19 has ravaged the country, most severely affecting nursing home residents, highly populated communities, and minorities. In the first three months of the pandemic, there were more than 1.6 million confirmed

Why is the United States the most severely impacted nation?

There are a number of factors why the United States has the highest number of reported cases—over 2 million as of June 23rd. One is that we have the infrastructure and funds to test a lot. The more people we test, the more cases we can identify. Second, we are the third most populated country in the world, second only to China and India, so we have more people who can be infected. New York State is larger and more densely populated than many European countries, so it is understandable that the state will have death and infection rates comparable to entire countries. Third, we have a medical system that can track deaths and attribute cause of death better than most others in the world.

cases and 100,000 deaths in the United States alone, approximating 1,100 deaths per day[91]. As of May, 315 million people have been affected by widespread stay-at-home orders[46] confining them to their homes except for essential trips and exercise. Infectious diseases experts have warned of resurgences as the economy opens up. As of this writing in early July, the number of COVID positive cases in the U.S. has surpassed 3 million and there have been more than 130,000 COVID related deaths.

Unemployment

The unemployment rate has soared to an unprecedented 18.6% of the labor force[63]. 39 million Americans applied for initial unemployment in the first nine weeks of the pandemic[61], with over 25 million claiming benefits[62]. This compares to 1.7 million claiming benefits during the same time last year[62]. Without seasonal adjustment, the raw number was 3.5 million Americans currently unemployed[61]. By early July, this number increased to 47 million Americans filing for unemployment[127]. Job loss predominantly affects poorer Americans, with 40% of low-income homes affected as compared to 19% of those earning between $40,000 and $100,000. As Americans lose their jobs, they save rather than spend, further damaging the economy. And loss of income results in reduced tax revenue to the government, making it more difficult to support stimulus packages to the people. Despite this economic devastation, President Trump stays optimistic, stating "Vaccine or no vaccine, we're back. And we're starting the process. We're going to have a really tremendous year next year. We're going to have a really good fourth quarter[64]."

Stimulus packages

On March 27th, President Trump signed the Coronavirus Aid, Relief, and Economic Security (CARES) Act, which provided a $2.2 trillion stimulus package[5]. This included $500 billion for distressed businesses, $350 billion for small business loans, $260 billion for expansion of the unemployment program, and $300 billion for direct stimulus payments to approximately 175 million Americans. Some small business payments went to larger companies such as Shake Shack, who chose to return the loans amidst backlash from consumers angry that the loans were inappropriately requested. The Aspen Institute think tank received negative attention for accepting an $8 million small business loan despite having a $115 million endowment and billionaires on its board.

The CARES Act has been the first of three economic stimulus packages (the third is being debated in Congress at this moment) and was the only to directly send stimulus checks to Americans. For many these stimulus checks were crucial to pay for bills and groceries after they lost their jobs or had a decrease in income. For most, it was not enough. In order to receive a stimulus check you had to have a social security number and a combined household income of less than $200,000. Democratic senators have proposed other bills that could provide hazard pay for essential workers, student loan forgiveness, and a basic monthly universal income. On May15th the House passed a $3.3 trillion relief package that would provide another round of direct stimulus payments to citizens[44]. It is doubtful the bill will be passed by the Senate. President Trump has called for Payroll Tax cuts to put more money in the hands of employers and workers. They Payroll Tax is a 15% tax typically split evenly between employers and employees. If you are self-employed, you incur all the burden of this tax. The revenues of this tax are used to fund Social Security payments.

Social Distancing

Director of the CDC Infectious Diseases Department, Dr. Anthony S. Fauci, was launched into the limelight as a prime expert on the coronavirus and a leader in America's efforts to control the virus. He has recommended strict social distancing measures from the start of the pandemic. Current social distancing guidelines recommend staying at home except for essential travel such as to the grocery or pharmacy or for exercise, maintaining 6 feet of social distance from other people, and wearing a mask. Social distancing has been successful in decreasing the number of cases at the peak of the epidemic, thereby preventing hospitals from being overwhelmed. Resurgences in cases are expected as we re-open the economy and could reach significant heights when coinciding with the flu season in the fall and winter.

Working from Home

Nearly half the U.S. workforce may now be working from home[80]. With saved commute time, increased work productivity, and the need for less office space, many have questioned whether work from home will be the new normal. Companies like Facebook, Google, and Apple have said their employees can choose to work from home for the rest of the year. My husband, parents, brother, and sister and brother in-law all worked from home during the pandemic, and their ability to do so was a great relief due to school closures. Other research-proven benefits of working from home are improved work/life balance, mental health, and reduced pollution[80] and cost of gasoline. The most common complaint I heard from telecommuters is that they miss seeing their co-workers. Many agree that their preferred situation in a post-pandemic world would be a combination of in-person and work-from-home days.

Sports

The worldwide sporting calendar was dramatically halted in response to COVID-19. No other event has caused such a tremendous disruption to sports since World War II. The 2020 Summer Olympics and Paralympics, due to take place in Tokyo, have been rescheduled, and the eleventh World Games have also been postponed. Sports are huge source of entertainment in the country. My younger brother, Josh Parasar, works for ScoreTrade--a live sports betting company. He tells me, "Sports is one of the industries that's been hurt most by the quarantine as teams worldwide have taken major cuts in valuation. ScoreTrade typically focuses on baseball, basketball, and football but has been hit by plummeting sports wagers, and has switched to eSports during the quarantine." Josh is a Yankees fanatic (Derek Jeter's 6 foot 3-inch profile hung outside his door throughout our childhood), and ardently hopes "that players and owners can put their egos aside and come to a profit sharing agreement that will allow partial seasons." Sports will soon start to reopen but without fans in the audience.

Some critics complain that if athletes can restart their seasons, albeit sans spectators, why can't gyms reopen? Arguably gyms could be a nidus for infection with people reusing equipment and in close proximity to each other. One gym owner in NJ defended his decision to reopen, stating "When are bills are due and our families are hungry, sitting and waiting is no longer an option." His gym was open for four days before being forced to shut it down by the state.

Prisons[100]

Prisons are a nidus for infections, and have been hit hard by COVID-19 given that inmates reside in close quarters. All but three states have suspended medical copays for inmates and many have initiated release of inmates to decrease risk of infection spread. NYC let out more than 1,100 inmates and may other states have followed suit. Of course, this may result in higher crime rates, especially in the setting of economic turmoil.

Elections

COVID-19 has halted several state elections due to fear of virus spread by in-person polling. The pandemic will have a huge impact on the November 2020 presidential elections, where approaches to re-opening the country will be a central issue[64]. Many states are currently offering absentee ballots to encourage voting while maintaining social distance.

Graduations

Many 2020 graduates, myself included, will have remote or drive-through graduation ceremonies. Celebrities have banded together to make these extra-special experiences, with Oprah Winfrey and others recording commencement addresses for graduates. Creative alternatives have been showcased across the country, with one high school posting large pictures of its graduate along its entry way. Our residency class will graduate over Zoom with many co-residents and faculty in attendance. While not ideal for many, the dedication of our program director and staff in making the event special is touching and memorable in itself. NY state is allowing "socially distant" graduations to take place starting on June 26th.[110]

Redeployed to the ED During the Pandemic

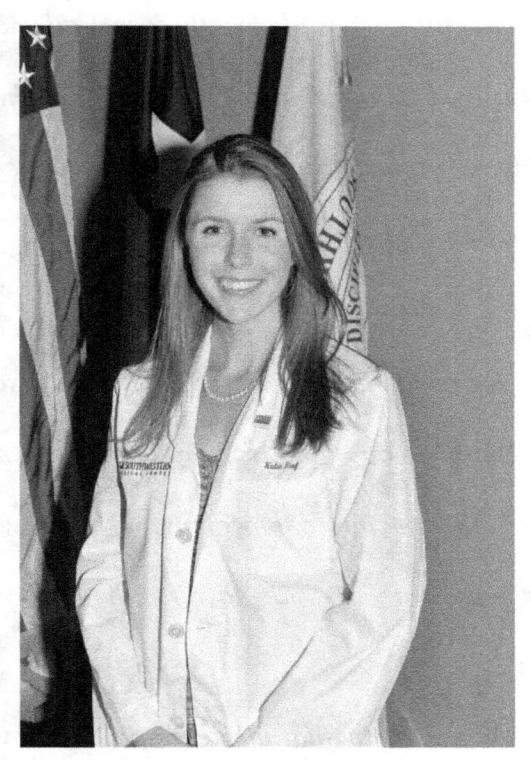

—*Dr. Katie Rief, MD, Physical Medicine & Rehabilitation Resident Physician, NYC*

When were you deployed to the ED? Mid-March.

What was it like to work in the emergency department at the epicenter of the pandemic? *The thing that was most striking was how quickly everyone could pivot and create this completely new infrastructure to see patients and pull in members of teams who were not necessarily emergency medicine trained. Of course, we were not going to automatically have the skill set of people who were particularly trained for this. But I think there is a lot of impressive versatility among our colleagues and at the leadership level to facilitate our redeployed staff's participation in a safe and effective manner. There were a lot of discussions early on when our program was deciding how many residents to redeploy, whether we should redeploy attendings, how is this all going to work. Some in our physiatry group were concerned that though we are specialists in musculoskeletal care, a large part of our practice is outpatient and we haven't been in a situation to treating acute illness as seen in the ED in this pandemic.*

Many were concerned that we would not be able to help in a direct way and that was completely disproven. I'm really proud of our colleagues for how we participated because everyone who was redeployed and put themselves in an uncomfortable position outside of their skill set was pleasantly surprised to see that we actually were very helpful members of the team. I think that not only attests to the hard work of our redeployed residents and faculty but also speaks about the receiving services and how incredibly helpful they were in guiding us and making us feel comfortable.

Were residents from other specialties also redeployed? *Yes, absolutely, there was urology, ophthalmology, surgery, physiatry, and anesthesia of course was instrumental. A big change was that the internal medicine residents who are typically rotating in the emergency department were redeployed to the ICUs, so we took their places.*

How was the camaraderie in the ED? *It was wonderful. We were welcomed with open arms as colleagues and equals. We couldn't ask for more appreciative hosts. They taught us how to function there and were a resource for questions.*

How did you determine which patients should be admitted and which should go home? *The most important determinants were vital signs and home support. We did not feel comfortable sending people who lived alone home. Vital sign cutoffs changed through the pandemic as capacity changed. Prior to the pandemic, you would admit someone who desaturates with exertion, but it became clear that if they admitted everyone at 92-93% saturation while walking, we would have no room for patients with resting hypoxia. There were some creative* *ways to deal with this and protocols that arose. Patients with good support at home and borderline saturations were discharged home with a pulse oximeter, follow up phone calls with ER staff at 24 and 48 hours and strict return precautions. Those who were at higher risk were sent home with supplemental oxygen with similar ER follow-ups. This allowed us to expand capacity for patients who were hypoxic at rest. It was a different way of approaching medicine since you're not used to sending someone desaturating home. We were more conservative with older patients and those who had comorbidities. For patients who you suspected did not have coronavirus, we wanted them to stay out of the hospital at all costs. It was often uncomfortable to send these patients home, but on a higher level you're trying to do what's best for the patient and it's most dangerous for them to be in the hospital.*

Which patients were tested? *A large percentage of the time I was in the ED there was not enough capacity for testing unless patients were being admitted to the hospital. Early on the policy was to only test patients who were admitted with COVID-19 symptoms, then it expanded to testing all admitted patients. As more swabs have become available and the ability to perform rapid antigen tests arose, there was an evolution to allow testing for even patients being discharged from the ED.*

Was there a high rate of burnout for providers working long shifts? *I think it was highly variable and a lot of people are doing some interesting work on healthcare provider strain. The reason it's so variable is because everyone has different stressors. I don't live with anyone at home so I wasn't concerned that I would be taking this home to anyone. My family lives in another state with low rates of coronavirus. I did everything recommended in terms of*

PPE and was fortunate to feel healthy throughout the time I worked there. For me, I found it to be a wonderful way to help and learn at the same time. These things contributed to a lack of burnout. Also working very reasonable hours—they still maintained the 80-hour work week for residents. You're tired after 80 hours a week but it's doable. I think some of the attendings and people working in positions with more personal responsibility were at higher risk for burnout. That being said, the people I worked directly with were very resilient on the surface and functioning very well in less than ideal circumstances.

What were some of the challenges you faced in taking care of ED patients? *In those early weeks where things were up in the air you could feel the intention and uncertainty of not knowing how bad it was going to get. We were doing everything we could, but you have no idea how much more it's going to escalate. Patients would say "I'm so scared to go home because I've heard with this disease you could get really sick out of the blue." And that's totally true and you don't really have anything to tell them. And I still struggle with that when patients are leaving rehab now after being asymptomatic for weeks now. Our best guess is that you can go home and won't infect your family members after you're been asymptomatic for weeks, but we don't really know."*

Have you been tested? *At this point I haven't since I haven't had any symptoms. It's not going to change my behavior—I'm going to continue to wear PPE, I'm going to continue to be careful. If they want to test me for knowledge regarding the number of people who have been exposed, I would be happy to do it. At this point, I don't see a benefit given the limited sensitivity of the tests available.*

Many of us at had symptoms early in February and many who have had significant exposure to the virus have had negative antibody tests. What do you think about the accuracy of the test? *I am skeptical about whether we really understand how the immune response works for this virus. A positive test is very helpful, but a negative test really isn't because what if you just didn't mount enough of an immune response to have a titer level that resulted in a positive response, or you didn't wait long enough before being tested for antibodies to be produced.*

For the past week, you have returned to the acute rehabilitation unit. How has that transition been? *After 8 weeks in the ER it is strange to go back to your normal circumstances. I've seen some of these patients when they were in extremis being admitted to our ED, and now, a month and a half later they are doing really well in our rehab unit! It's satisfying but also eye opening in showing how much we are going to have to deal with moving forward. One of the things that we are all seeing is a large percentage of patients with peripheral nerve injuries, which could be from prolonged critical illness, proning and positioning, or an effect of the virus.*

Are there any patient experiences that most impacted you? *One of the hardest thing in the ER was communicating with family members who were not there. You end up introducing yourself to someone and in the next breath, asking about end of life wishes, which is such a terrible way to start a conversation. And as much as you would want to build rapport and to get to know this person, it's not always possible when there's an immediate need to ask "Do* *you want your loved one to be intubated? Do you want them to be resuscitated?" We got more comfortable with it over time, and of course the emergency doctors who do this on a daily basis were much more skilled at it. And I think one of the nice things was that our palliative care colleagues set up teaching tools regarding how to make those conversations flow better, and also offered their skills to offload the ER doctors' role. When you're managing six different crashing patients, you don't really have time to sit down and have a great goals of care discussion- as much as you want to, it's not going to happen. The palliative care team volunteered to be involved with that and they were great. They really stepped up to the plate and helped with many difficult patient conversations.*

What patient demographic did you typically see? *The vast majority of patients were older. The general trends that have been reported in the media have been accurate in my experience. Patients over 60 are at very high risk, but there were a lot patients who came in quite sick who were only 40 or 50. The difference is that the younger are much more likely to survive even if intubated.*

Did you find any interventions other than oxygen supplementation to be helpful? *I don't think any pharmaceuticals helped, other than helping the doctors feel like we were doing something. Though we really don't have the data or well-conducted research to definitively say what helps and what doesn't quite yet. Proning was actually very impressive to me. We don't have a great clinical trial to show its efficacy in COVID patients yet, but I thought that awake proning was one of the most interesting ideas, because it makes cognitive sense that if you have people lie on their stomachs before they are intubated this may help. I* *saw several people that were desaturating on multiple layers of oxygen, but after they rolled onto their stomachs, they popped up! Effective and relatively low risk.*

What would you like people to know about COVID-19? The mortality may be low when you look of the numbers who actually died, but different parts of the country, and even different parts of Manhattan, deal with different morality rates because of physical proximity and difficulties social distancing. So the challenges we face here in NYC are different than in other parts of the country. You hear people in New York saying "We are getting slammed, we are so overwhelmed" and you see people in California saying "We are waiting for the surge. It's not here yet [This has changed since this interview was conducted]." I think a one-size fits-all policy for moving forward is not the best strategy. It needs to be individualized to the local environment. Ultimately the virus is very dangerous and we have seen first-hand how it can overwhelm the healthcare system, so I think it's unrealistic for people to dismiss it and go back to normal. That being said, on the other side, we have a group of people that is so immersed in what has happened in NYC that they want to apply the strategies we have used here for a really conservative re-opening that is in my opinion appropriate for a large population-dense city like New York, but may not be applicable to other regions of the country. The fact that this has become a political divide is concerning to me because it shouldn't be a political decision whether we re-open or we close, it should be a local decision tailored to the surrounding environment. One of the most important things we can do is to share knowledge with our colleagues across the country. If this starts to happen to you, here is the way you can logistically expand capacity, here is how to rearrange teams, here is how we cross-trained our physicians and nurses. This is what works and this is what doesn't.

Having that information puts you so much farther ahead, because that's part of what took so long and was so challenging and so scary. It's not about stockpiling millions of masks for a crisis that may never come. It's about if we do need them, how we obtain them quickly.

Why do you think New York was hit so hard? *I think it's a combination of factors—the population density, the patient demographics, and the fact that it is such an international travel hub. It's hard to know exactly and there are many people studying this. But before things were brought to light, so many people came into New York that were probably infectious. That many people never would have gone to North Dakota, and even if they did, they wouldn't be living in apartment rooms right next to each other, passing on the subway, passing on the street, allowing for that infectious spread. There have been a lot of criticisms of hospital capacity, saying we should have had more ICU beds, we should have had more hospital beds, we knew this crisis was coming. I don't think that's a fair criticism because when you're not in crisis for most of the decade, those beds would sit empty. I think it goes back to structuring a supply chain to be pushed into action when you need it. I think at baseline our hospital has 300 ICU beds and they expanded to 900 in 19 days—it was really impressive.*

Is there anything else you would like to add? *Overall, it was such a privilege to get to work in that environment, and I'm so thankful for my time there and getting to be a part of what will be a major part of New York and world history. It was a huge opportunity to learn and expand my skill set and really contribute.*

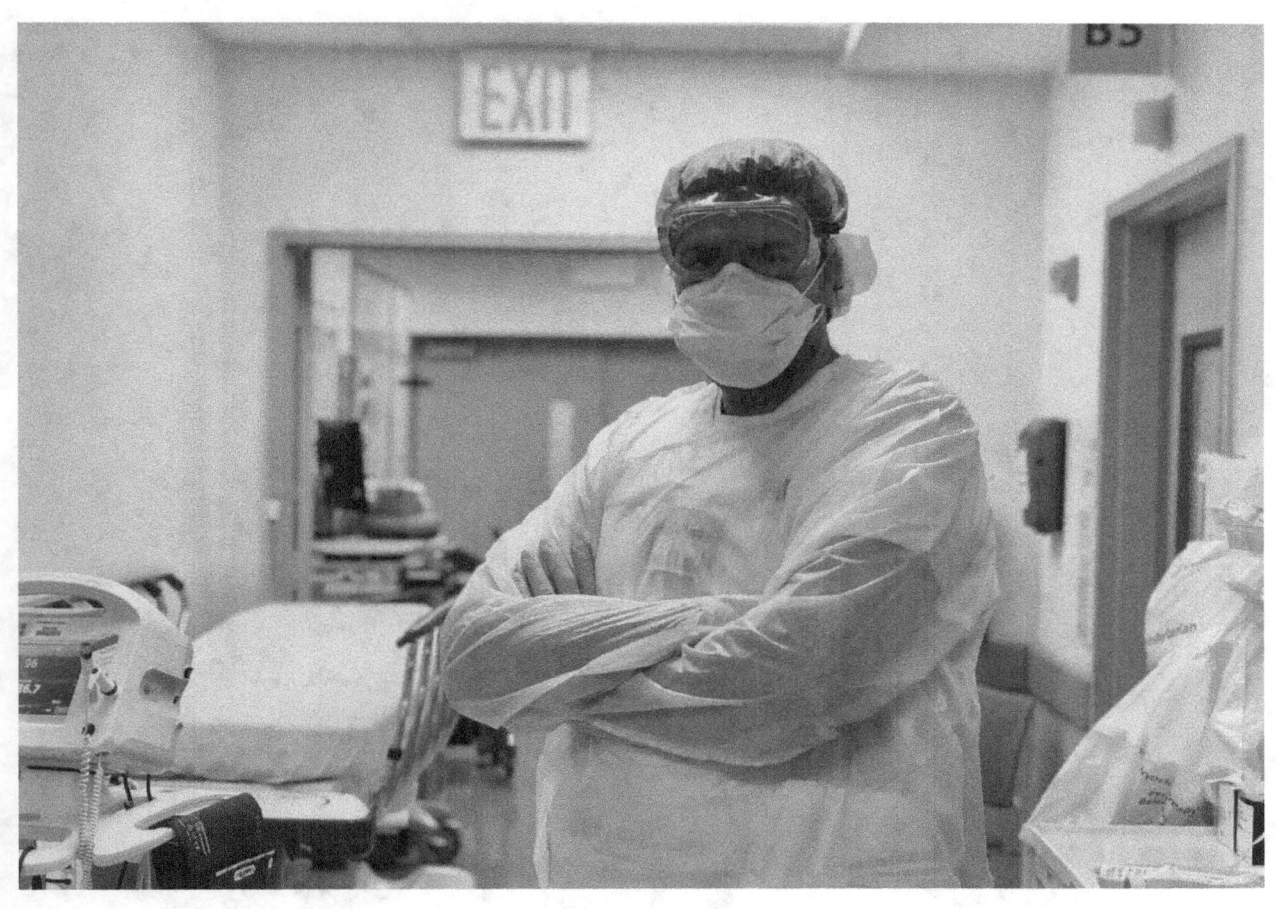

"I became a nurse because I enjoy helping others. I'm proud to be a part of this wonderful team in the ED. I couldn't picture myself doing anything else but emergency nursing. Together we can overcome this just like anything else.

- RJ Bharath, Registered Nurse, Emergency Department, NYC

International Perspective:

Ramat Hashofet, Israel

—Ronen Benhaim

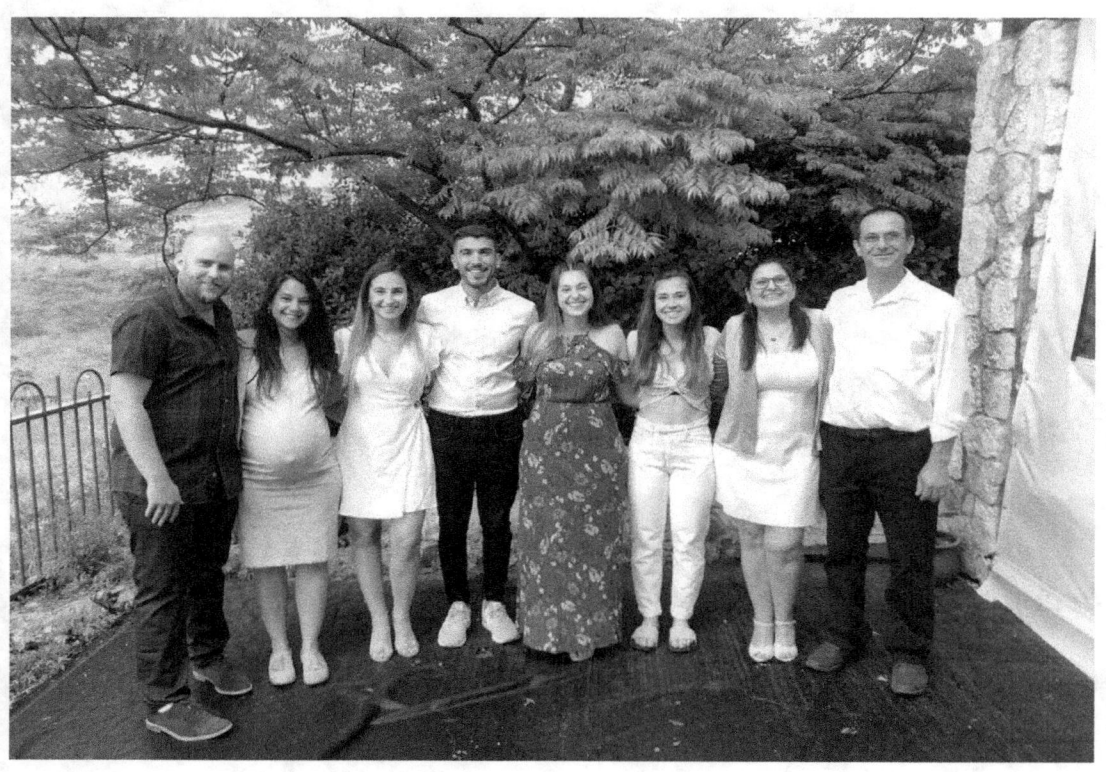

My name is Ronen Ben Haim, I'm from Israel, married to Murielle. We have 4 daughters & 1 grandson. We live in Kibbutz Ramat Hashofet at the north of Israel. I'm VP sales of a small Israeli startup and my wife is a community nurse.

How has the pandemic affected you personally and professionally? *Starting January of 2020 we came to know of "the Corona" (how we refer to the pandemic in Israel). By the end of January, our government stopped all incoming flights from Asia (we may be one of the first countries to do so, and this gave us more time to be prepared for the peak of the virus).*

During February, some of the Diamond Princess cruise passengers were Israeli families so the Corona became the headline news. Israelis from all over the world started to make their ways "back home" to acknowledge the fact that Israel is a safe place.

In March, our government started to close public places, including schools, synagogues, mosques, and churches so most of us couldn't go to work. By the end of March our country was on lock down and only critical work was allowed. Others could only go out for medical care or home supply. It was emphasized that families not visit their elderly family members. My wife is a nurse and had to go to work, performing her duty amidst the ever-changing protocol and facing supply shortages like other countries around the world. At our company, the last week of March was very black. Customer after customer started to call to inform us of business closures, especially in retail. We sent our employees on unpaid vacation during which they received Social Security benefits.

From our family perspective, fortunately our eldest daughter lives with us in a separate living unit, so we enjoyed great quality time with her and our 1 year old grandson. We know this is something that many grandparents couldn't do.

How has Israel been affected by the pandemic? *In the first phase Israel was leading as one of the safe countries worldwide. As we are "an island", we stopped international flights early. Fortunately, and unfortunately, we as a country know how to deal with emergencies—wars* *continually have an impact on the civilian population—and we passed the first phase of the Corona pandemic relatively well. Our total death totaled 300 people with roughly 15,000 infected by the virus. This along with the social activities of thousands of volunteers created a very good feeling of being an Israel at the Israeli state.*

What are your thoughts regarding how your Israel handled the pandemic? *The first phase was relatively successful, especially with comparison to worldwide numbers. The growing civilian pressure to reopen the "full life"/ market has led us to move dramatically fast into the second phase. In the last few weeks there is a great growing anger at our government over two major points:*

1) Failing to set up mass infrastructure to manage the medical tests, provide fast results, update patients, manage the epidemiology investigations, and to be able to analyze the results so that life and economic decisions are being made based on true facts.

2. Economic situation: our financial support programs are "too late, too small," leading families into great financial problems with fears for the future.

The fact that we moved into the second phase with growing numbers of impacted/ isolated people, has led to re-close most of the entertainment industry: couture, wedding, pubs, etc.

Most of us feel the following sentiment towards our government: "We followed all your instructions, we gave you two months to prepare medically and economically and to provide us basic needs, and you failed on your part.

Another major factor is that in March we went through a third election process after no one could set up a coalition and our prime minister Bibi Netanyahu is in the middle of a lawsuit. Thus, our geopolitics & security is very sensitive at this time.

Any final thoughts? *We are in a great crisis, and the world after Corona will be totally different due to the great toll on our economy. Israel is a relatively young, smart country and has an opportunity to move out of the crisis but this will take time until then we will have a lot of negatively impacted people.*

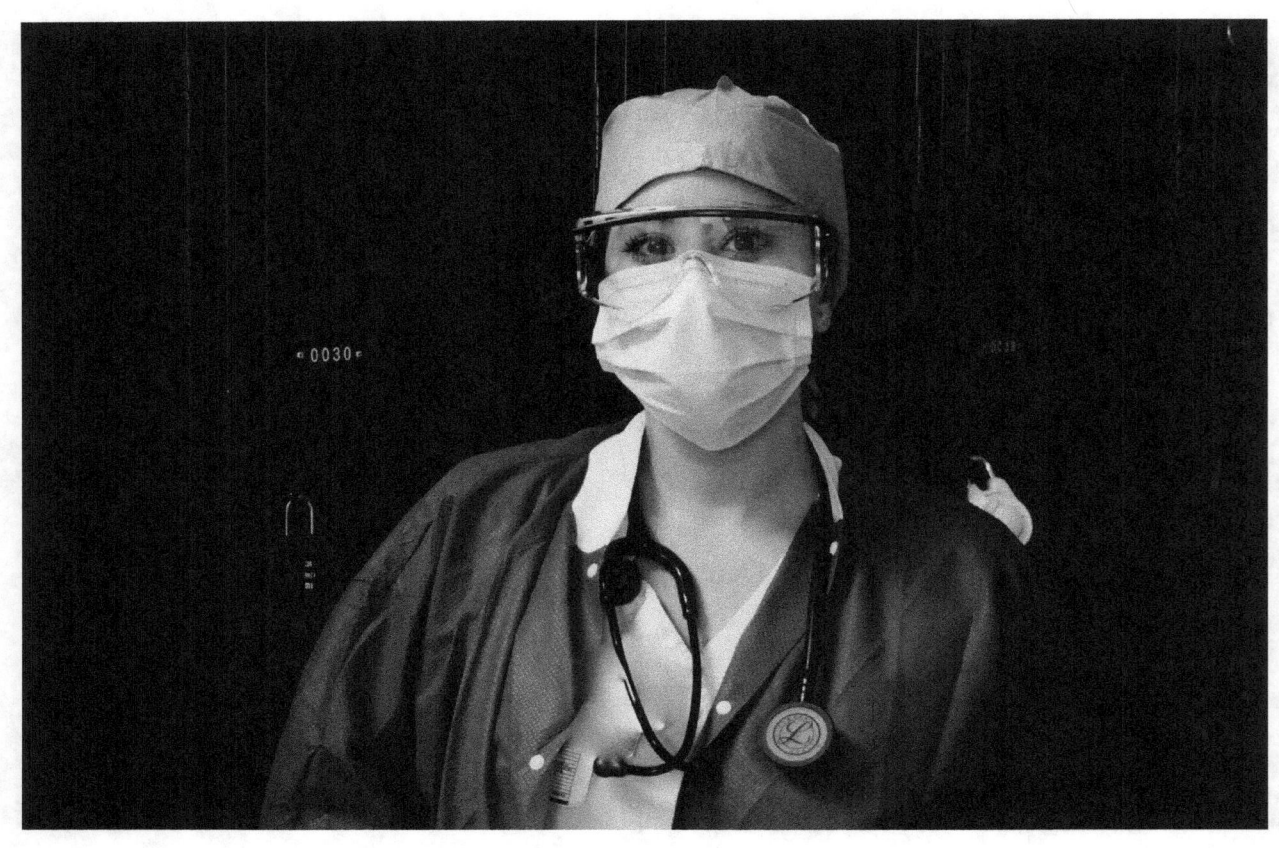

"There's nowhere else I'd rather be than on the frontline fighting this virus. COVID-19 has brought on the darkest days imaginable, but it has also brought out the best in people. To my community, here and afar, the donations, cheers, prayers, and messages of hope- you make showing up worth it."

-Lauren Laguna, Registered Nurse, Emergency Department, NYC

CHAPTER 17: RE-OPENING AMERICA

"We cannot let the cure be worse than the problem itself. At the end of the 15 day period, we will make a decision as to which way we want to go!

-President Donald J. Trump

After the April peak, COVID-19 cases in the U.S. started to steadily wane. Nevertheless, governors have been cautious to re-open their states in fear of resurgence. By the beginning of May more than 2/3 of states have started to relax their restrictions due to economic pressures[47], and by the week of May 18th all 50 states are in the process of gradually re-opening. Only 3% of the population has been tested, so it is still difficulty to accurately calculate the prevalence of the disease. Fauci has stated that Americans would experience "needless suffering and death" if the country reopened too early[6]. He made an appeal to the Senate to prevent premature opening of the country, arguing that this "would actually set us back on our quest to return to normal." Rick Bright, who was the former director of the Biomedical Advanced Research and Development Authority, has also stated that "without clear planning and implementation of the steps that I and other experts have outlined, 2020 will be the darkest winter in modern history."

Kentucky Senator Rand Paul has criticized Dr. Fauci, stating that case numbers have been overestimated and that we should look for guidance from other countries with more lenient lockdowns that have still managed to slow the spread of COVID-19 while keeping their economies open. Sweden is a classic example—the European country was unique in its handling of COVID-19, as one of the few countries who did not enforce quarantine of its citizens. Paul advocates for an individualized school district by school district approach to reopen the economy.

President Trump has defended America's approach to reopening the country. He has largely left the decision to reopen up to the states since some parts of the country have been hit harder than others. The White House has issued guidelines for a three-phase reopening based on the recommendations of public health experts[133].

Protests erupted throughout the country as unemployed workers exercised their First Amendment right to demand that the country be reopened as soon as possible. They argued that strict lockdown orders were an infringement upon their constitutional rights and that the government's quarantine was ruining the livelihood of small businesses around the country. In Michigan, protestors gathered outside the state capitol building during a session where lawmakers were voting on whether to extend to the lockdown—they ruled to re-open. Many citizens criticize the protestors—who often do not wear masks and are noncompliant with social distancing—for putting more people at risk by encouraging the spread of the disease. Current polls report that more people are afraid of the economy reopening too soon than an extended lockdown, with 2 out of 3 Americans feeling that gatherings of more than 10 people would still be unsafe by July.

Georgia was one of the first states to re-open. On April 24th, Governor Kemp announced the reopening of hair, nail, and tattoo salons. Three days later this was extended to theatres, restaurant dine-in service, and private social clubs, and allowed the scheduling of essential elective surgeries. Services that remained closed included bars, nightclubs, amusement park rides, and live performance venues. Tennessee and Florida were the next states to follow Georgia's lead.

More severely hit areas such as NYC and Washington D.C. extended their lockdowns through June 6th and 8th respectively, while other less affected parts of NY and Maryland started to open in mid-May. California, while not hit as hard as some other states, has also extended its restrictions.

By mid-June, 22 states have experiences spikes in COVID-19 states during the re-opening process. In several states, the rates of new cases are the highest they have been during the pandemic. The country is conflicted over whether we are re-opening too soon and will cause more deaths in doing so, or whether we may be costing more lives and economic devastation due to continued lockdown and neglect of other illnesses. There is no clear-cut answer and as the situation differs significantly in each state and city, a one-size-fits-all approach to re-opening may not be effective.

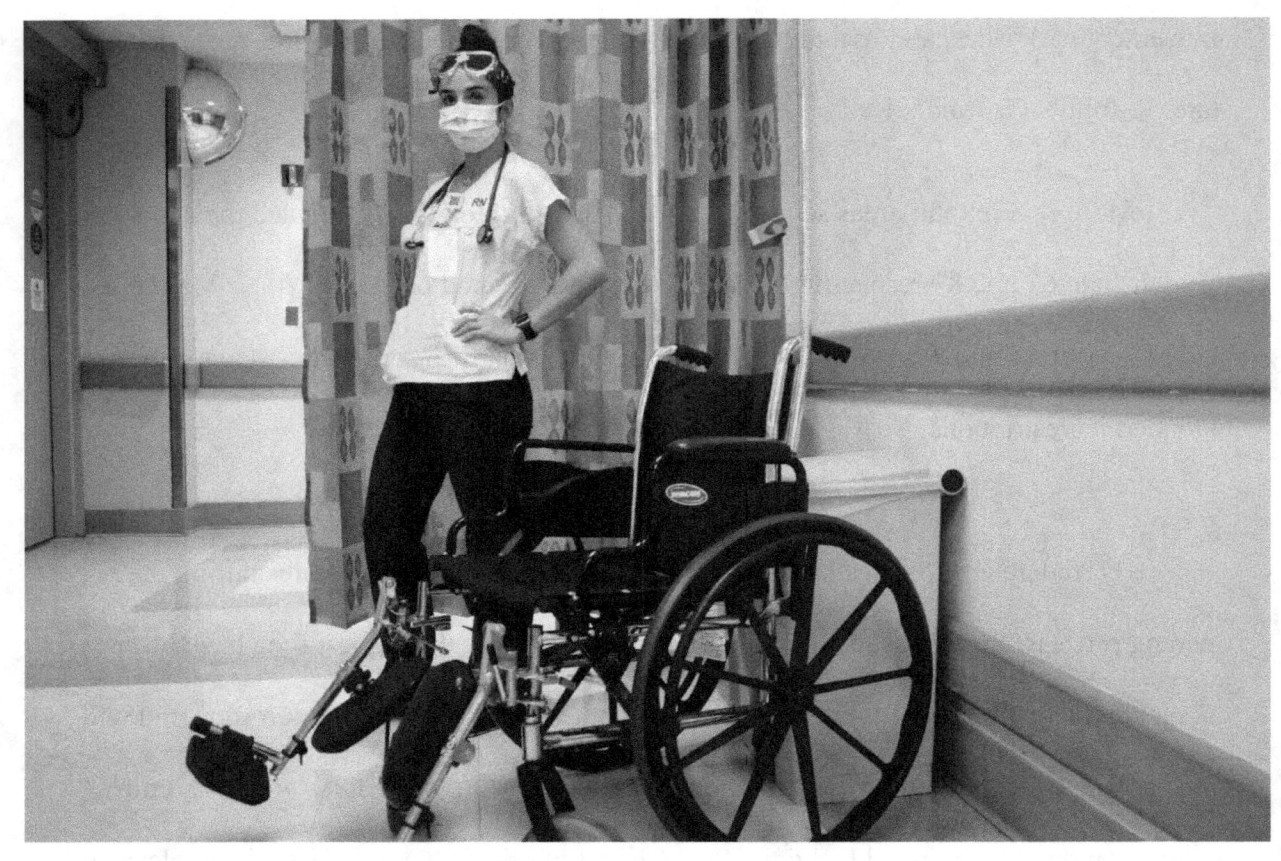

"Nursing truly is a job like no other and the day it became my reality was one of the most memorable days of my life. I would've never imagined that I'd be working through a global pandemic on the frontlines but this is what it's all about. To say the team I get to work beside is amazing would be an absolute understatement and I don't think I could do this without them. I know I speak for us all when I say, please just do your part and stay home. This will end and it

won't be easy, but it's up to us to flatten the curve. I can't wait for this to be a distant memory and to give everyone I love the biggest hug they've ever received and make sure they know just how important they are. I'm thankful that this has taught me to cherish the little things and never take anything in this life for granted. Shout out to my ED crew, we have a lot of social distancing to make up for when this is all over. Love you all."

-Nicole Labarr, Registered Nurse, Emergency Department, NYC

Caring for Geriatric Patients During the Pandemic

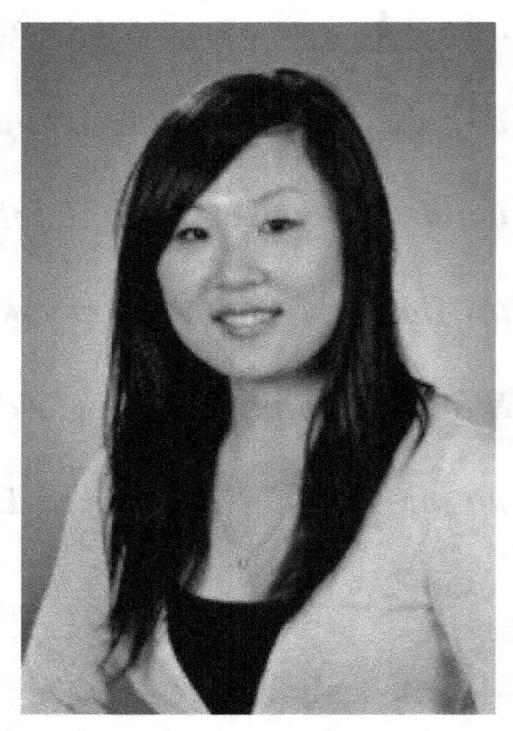

-Dr. Gina Kang, MD, Geriatric Fellow at Yale New Haven Hospital, CT

What was your experience caring for geriatric patients during the pandemic? *A majority of my time was working in the geriatric inpatient unit during this time since this is where I was needed. Despite being a "COVID-negative unit," we were still greatly impacted by the pandemic. There were several challenges that affected patient care, especially in our older adults. First off, discharge planning was very difficult since a lot of facilities were closed to accepting patients or had strict admission criteria. Many of our older adult patients were essentially living in the hospital, while waiting for a safe discharge plan. Very valid and real concerns were raised by family and patients who were unsafe to go home, but did not want to go to a short-term rehab or skilled nursing facility because they were afraid that if they went to a facility, they would die from COVID. Other challenges included social isolation, taking extra precautions with our more vulnerable population, and assessing atypical or asymptomatic presentations of COVID in older adults. Being in the hospital was especially hard on our older patients who had cognitive impairment or dementia. It is a pretty scary place to be alone, especially in the hospital with people you don't know while you're sick and add a pandemic on top of that.*

What was it like for your patients to have no visitors? Several of my patients have dementia and were unable to understand why their families weren't visiting them. It was the toughest thing and made me really sad. It's so important for our patients, especially those with dementia to see familiar faces. This helps make the environment less confusing, improve orientation, and helps to motivate engagement in therapy and treatments. I remember one of my patients who was scared, confused, and anxious wondering why his family wasn't coming. He thought he had done something to upset them and I had to remind him that this wasn't the case, it broke my heart. The nurse and I would try to sit with him and talk, but obviously we are not the same as having a loved one there.

Did you see an increase in mental health disorders? I definitely saw an increase in mental health disorders such as an increase in anxiety and depressive symptoms. The social isolation with no visitors and seclusion, really had a toll on my patients. This affected their motivation to engage in their treatment management plans such as physical and occupational therapy or even getting out of bed to a chair. This also took a toll on family and caretakers as they were unable to be there for their loved ones. Though there were positive solutions provided by the hospital for communication, such as iPads for video conference, this was often unable to be utilized considering some of the capabilities were unavailable or our older patients had spouses or other family members who had a harder time utilizing these technological modalities. I can only imagine how emotionally stressful and terrifying it is to have a loved one in the hospital and are unable to be there. As much as we try to support our patients and be there for them, we are not their family and they need their loved ones, especially while they are sick and in the hospital.

Next year you will be starting a fellowship in palliative and hospice care. How has the pandemic changed your views of your future career path? Through this pandemic, it has *made me appreciate this field even more and how much palliative care has helped to support patients, families and other health care providers and how essential it is in providing comprehensive care and understanding what matters most to patients and families. I am so thankful to have this opportunity to do this fellowship and train under the very best.*

Is there anything you would like people to know about COVID-19? *It's real. I feel like every time I went into the hospital it was going into the unknown. It's such a scary time to be in the hospital for patients and providers. But I am so happy to be working alongside my colleagues and to be there for my patients. Everyone has been so amazing and banded together through this. It has made me so proud to be a part of this healthcare team.*

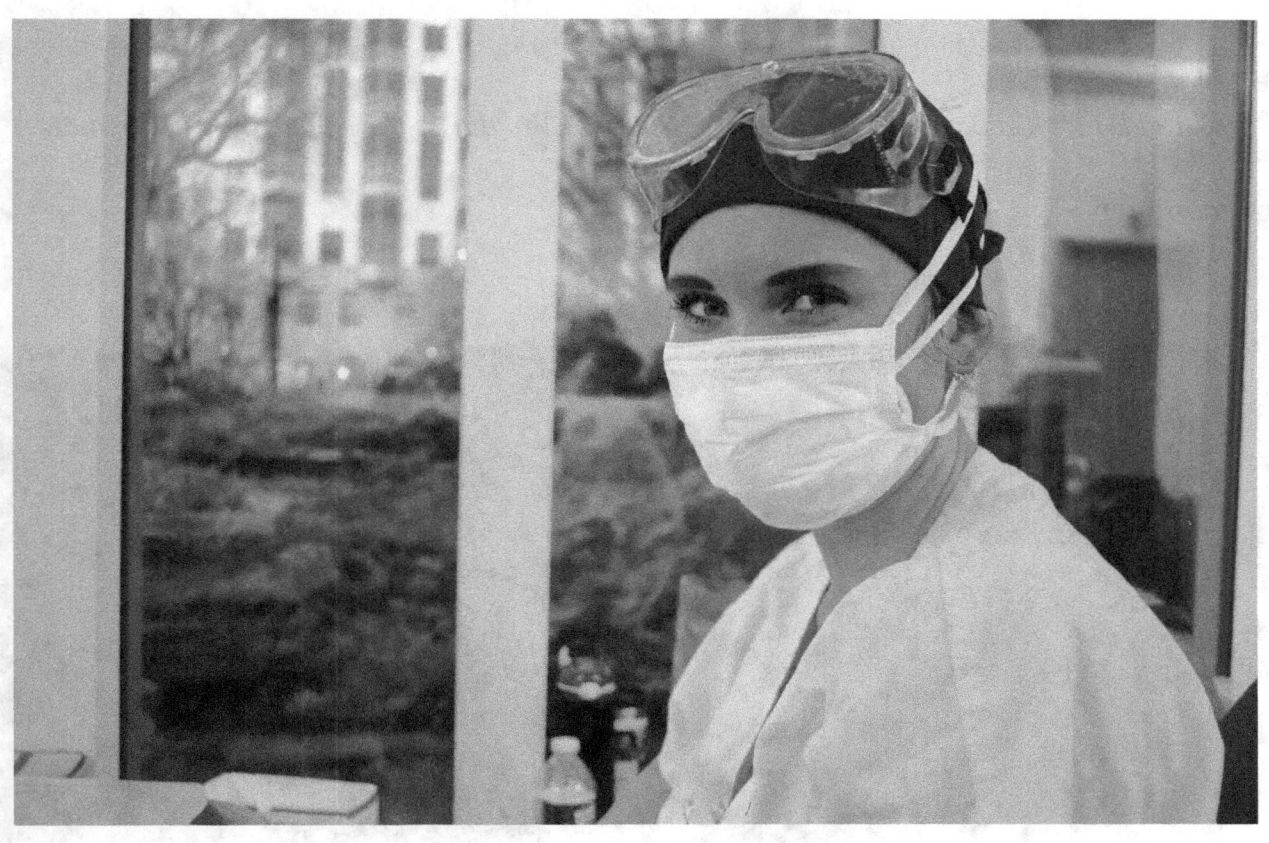

"[The patients'] families can't be with them at the bedside to comfort them at this time due to the danger of the virus. But we can—and I consider that a privilege."

-Bridget Morrissey, Registered Nurse, Emergency Department, NYC

International Perspective: Helsinki, Finland

—*Pekka Pajamo, Chief Financial Officer of Varma, a large pension insurance company*

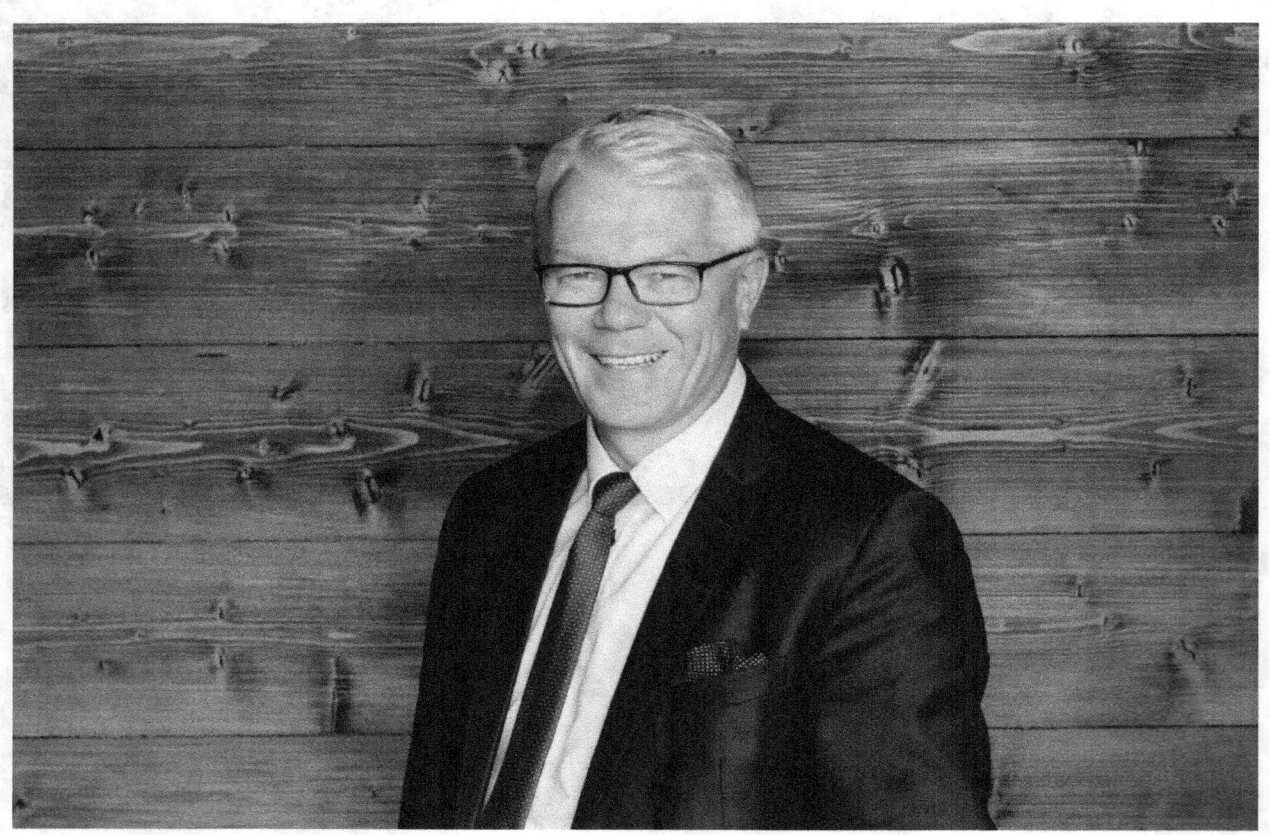

How has the pandemic affected you personally and professionally?

Professionally: Varma oversees pension related matters of over 900,000 persons in Finland. Every month, we pay pensions to some 340,000 persons, and for most, these pensions are *their sole source of income. Therefore, it is of utmost importance that our business continues in all circumstances. This is also of one of our legislative tasks.*

I am in charge of our business continuity and responsible for all preparations against any threats our business may have. We started our communications regarding the pandemic in early February, by providing our personnel with updated information regarding travelling abroad, restricting outside meetings, and also restricting meetings with visitors on our premises. This also included a strong suggestion of working from home and thus securing our own offices to be a non-corona place.

In mid-March, following orders given by our government, we ordered everyone to start working from home. The office has been literally empty after that. In June, we allowed personnel to return should they have difficulties working at home, such as small children, that may restrict them from concentrating on their work.

Practically all meetings, be it external or internal, have been arranged through net. Our effectiveness has grown, and people have been very satisfied with the approach we took (to ensure that the offices will remain clean and safe). The IT networks have worked fine and we have been able to move all our work to home offices.

We are returning to our offices in August. We have divided our workforce into two, with permission to come to the office every other week. This also ensures that the two groups do not meet. We will assess the progress of this method in August, and also strictly follow the guidance from the government of Finland.

Personally: First and foremost, my family has stayed safe and healthy all the time. This is of great importance. I happened to be travelling in Italy in the last week of February with the family. Once back in Finland, we ended up in a two weeks guarantee, even though there were no COVID-19 contaminations in Finland at that time. After the two weeks, I went back to the office for another week and then we closed our office, as described earlier.

My work has been dominated by the pandemic and our response to it. This has meant long hours in net meetings, contacting authorities, talking with colleagues in other companies, and almost daily net meetings with our management team. I am also the chairman for a body that co-ordinates all business continuity issues with social security insurance in Finland. This has provided in a true insight look into what government thinks, how they react and what is assumed from us.

As the Chairman of the Board of Directors of The Finnish National Theatre I have been deeply involved in handling the situation with close co-operation with the General Director and his team. Unfortunately, by the order of our government, we had to close all stages and cancel all performances for the spring season. The same had to be done also with The Finnish National Opera and Ballet where I am a board member.

As Finland is now more or less closed for the summer holidays, my thoughts are moving towards a safe start of work in August, in all areas of activity. It will be very interesting to see what the autumn has reserved for us. The global news at the moment is worrying, implying a second wave in the countries that were hit early, while the first wave still going strong in countries like USA and Brazil.

How has your country been affected? Finland is a country with a population of some 5.8 million. We have, for historical reasons, national legislation that under certain circumstances gives the authorities very large rights for restricting things like a pandemic to spread. This legislation was taken into use of in latter part of March 2020. Finland also has very high-quality social security and healthcare. There are no barriers in receiving care, if needed, and all residents are entitled to this care.

The most southern part of Finland, around Helsinki, where most people live, was closed for three weeks to all traffic. This slowed the spreading of the pandemic dramatically. The borders have been practically closed since March and only this week the Finns will be able to travel to some 26 countries. This has also reduced the risk of getting the virus from abroad and infecting other people.

In our hospitals, non-emergency care was postponed, and major resources were dedicated to treat those who were at risk of being infected with the virus. Intensive care units and seats are scarce, and they were reserved to treat virus related matters. So far, the system has worked fine, and the actions taken by the authorities have proved to be right.

As of today, there is a total of 7,295 persons that have caught the virus. Over the last 7 days, 38 new people have caught the virus, and 48 new persons in the 7 days before that. There are only 6 people under hospital care at the moment, and 329 persons have died of corona.

As for the economy, the closure of businesses has meant layoffs in practically almost all fields. Restaurants and bars were closed for the months of April and May, and allowed to open with 50 % capacity only in June. Take-away food has been popular, as well as people cooking at home. Many of the business are predicting a difficult autumn, as there is no certainty when business will pick up.

If you feel comfortable sharing, what are your thoughts regarding how your country handled the pandemic? The Finnish government's central goal was to flatten the curve of the virus. It was understood early in the process that managing that curve will leave time for the healthcare system to prepare for the larger scale pandemic and thus to treat those infected in a proper manner.

It is my understanding that this is the very thing that the Finnish government succeeded in doing properly. Although no death is acceptable, the hospital systems were not overwhelmed. Also, the restrictions set on businesses and public events and movement have proved to be successful.

The government has used large public funding to support businesses, healthcare, and public services. In the coming years, it will face major challenges in supporting economic growth and controlling levels of taxation. It is currently estimated that the Finnish economy will be the slowest within EU countries to recover from this pandemic.

Any final thoughts? One of the main characteristics of the pandemic has been that – as it is in the current world – all news travel fast. This is true to both actual news and rumours. Literally all people who have access to internet have also had access to current information on the pandemic as well its progress. I sincerely hope that this rather helped the fight against the virus instead of making it more difficult.

Many countries have put utmost effort into fighting the virus. In monetary terms this has meant more spending on each individual case (calculated as total spending divided by those infected or those who have lost their lives) than under normal circumstances in any health-related matter. At one stage, there was a discussion on this topic. I trust that once the pandemic is under control, the discussion will resume. Then we will most likely see arguments supporting the high spending as well as criticizing it. To all individuals, the value of human life should be the highest priority. We will only see later if the COVID-19 pandemic will change our thinking and our values.

CHAPTER 18:

ECONOMIC IMPACT IN AMERICA

"Disease impact would also ripple through the economy to disastrous effect. With everyone from air traffic controllers to truck drivers out sick, just-in-time inventory systems would crash, supply chains would collapse, for lack of some part production lines would shut down, while schools and day-care facilities might close for weeks, and an overburdened "last mile" would limit the ability of people to work from home."

-John M. Barry in the 2018 afterword to *The Great Influenza*, predicting the economic effects of a future pandemic

The unemployment rate rapidly escalated to 14.7% as companies deemed nonessential were forced to close. U.S. economy has shrunk nearly 40% in the second quarter[121]—levels not seen since the Great Depression. In the most heavily impacted areas, lines of people and cars have become a common sight, as unemployed workers waited to collect food for their families. The $8 trillion toll on the U.S. economy is expected to extend into the decade[97].

Chairman of the Federal Reserve, Jerome Powell, has declared that the economy will likely experience a long and painful recession, He states that the coronovarius pandemic is "the biggest shock our economy has felt in modern times[21]." Business leaders fear a protracted recession, surge in bankruptcies, high levels of youth unemployment, and an increase in cyberattacks as people work from home[58]. And with the country's mounting deficit there is the question, how will we pay for all this?

> *What is the difference between a depression and a recession?*[92]
>
> A recession describes two quarters of declining GDP. A depression is a prolonged recession (the timeline is not defined).

As millions of Americans have cancelled travel plans[127], airlines and travel companies like Airbnb were hit hard. Airbnb let go of more than 150 employees. The airline industry required a $50 billion bailout from the federal government.

Restaurants were initially asked to observe social distancing practices, limiting occupancy and proximity of diners. That changed to allowing only take-out and drive-through options, severely diminishing revenues and causing some restaurants to close. Some Asian American restaurants reported a declining customer base as early as January, as fear mounted regarding the novel Coronavirus discovery in China[46].

Many companies have had to close or file bankruptcy due to the virus. Payless plans to close more than 2,500 stores, Gymboree will close 800; department stores J.C. Penney, Neiman Marcus, and Stage Stores are filing for bankruptcy protection[40]. J.C. Penney, founded in 1913, employed approximately 90,000 employees in 846 department stores in February[40]. It survived the Great Depression, but not COVID-19. While department stores have been hit hard by the advent of online selling, COVID-19 has been the final blow as malls have shut down and brands are selling directly to consumers via online shopping[40]. Disney is expected to lose a whopping $1 billion in the quarter ending in June[132].

Even companies that you think may be doing better in the pandemic, such as Amazon and hospitals, are instead facing losses due to decreased revenue. Many outpatient physicians' practices have a significant reduction in patients as they must comply with social distancing laws and have a decreased demand from patients scared to leave their homes. While telemedicine visits have increased, many patients do not have the capability or desire to participate in these kind of visits, and so revenue has significantly decreased.

As homes fail to sell and vacation rentals go unoccupied, housing market prices are expected to plummet this summer due to supply for homes outstripping demand[41]. Furthermore, Oxford Economics predicts that 15% of homeowners will fall behind on their mortgage payments, which would result in more delinquencies than seen in the Great Recession[41]. Prior to the lockdown, the housing and vacation rental markets were booming[42]. The federal government is trying to spur demand by offering reduced mortgage rates for home-buyers; this is being discussed as part of the 3rd stimulus package in Congress right now.

As people lose jobs and face economic uncertainty, consumer spending has precipitously declined so even those businesses that have remained open are suffering[97]. Stimulus checks appeared to spur spending, with national retailers noting increased purchases during the weeks that the checks were released.

COVID-19 has redefined who is an essential worker. Whereas first line responders and healthcare workers generally receive esteem and respect, the virus has brought out the importance of grocery workers, mail carriers, food and agricultural workers, and those in transportation and public works. Many of these people never signed up for exposure to a deadly virus, and yet have kept our economy and way of life going through their hard work and dedication.

I am so thankful that I was able to work every day during the pandemic. Second to loss of life and medical morbidity, economic devastation has been one of the most heart-wrenching consequences. In a couple of months people have lost their hard-earned businesses, their ways of life—for many, their reasons to get up in the morning. In the hospital system where we have job security and we live and breathe the devastating health effects of the virus, we become blindsided to the destruction of people's financial security and life purpose around the world. There is no easy answer. Life is invaluable. But so is quality of life, and the lockdown has destroyed that for many people. Just as those of us who haven't been sick or had a loved one succumb to COVID can't fully appreciate the horror of the disease, those of us who have retained our livelihoods and financial security cannot fully understand the distress of not being able to work and provide for one's family. I echo the wisdom of Dr. Katie Rief, who counsels that decisions to re-open the country be made on a local basis, since each community has been impacted so differently. Instead of political rivalry, we must work together to maximize life as well as prioritize livelihood.

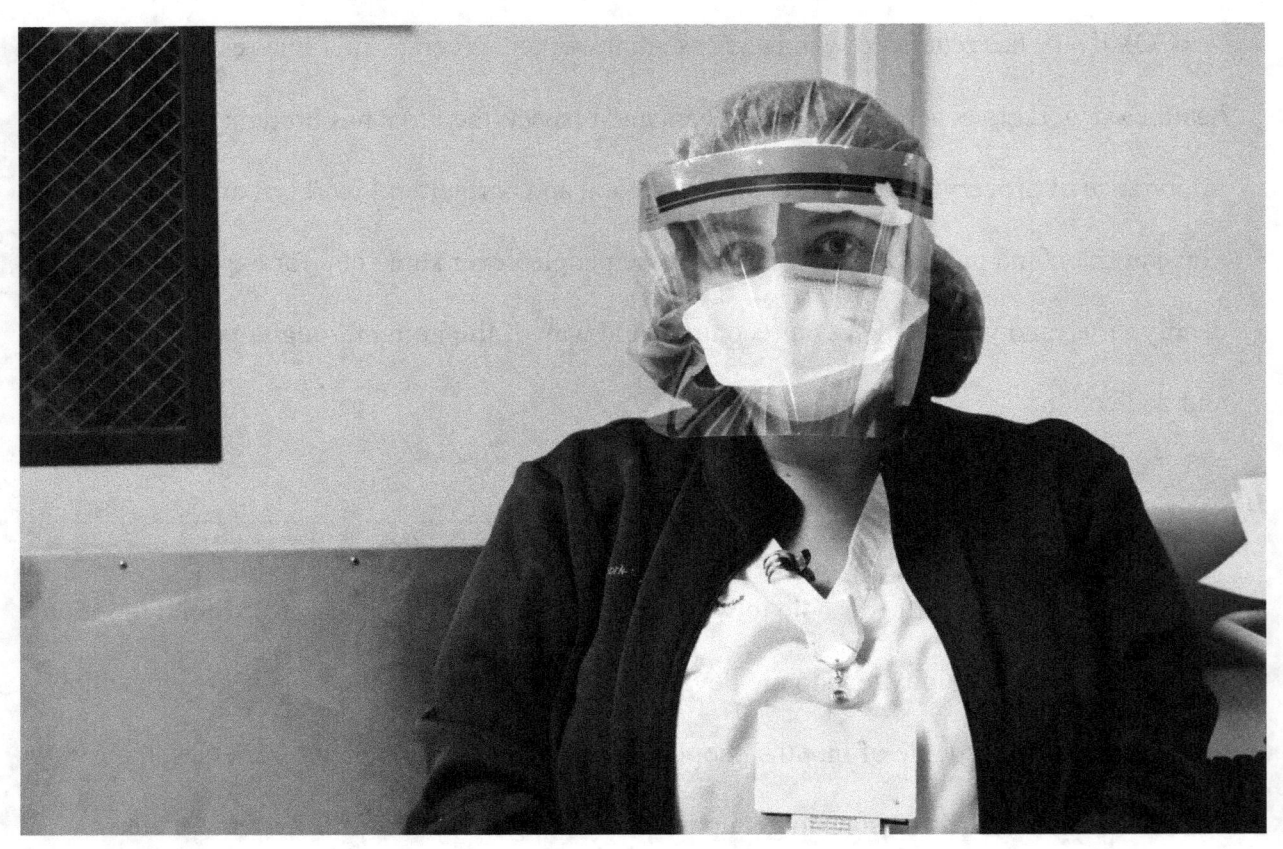

"I am here and I will always be here."

- Kaitlin Lucke, Registered Nurse, Emergency Department, NYC

Testing and Immunity

- Dr. Madhuri Tarumandas, MD, Infectious Diseases Specialist, NYC

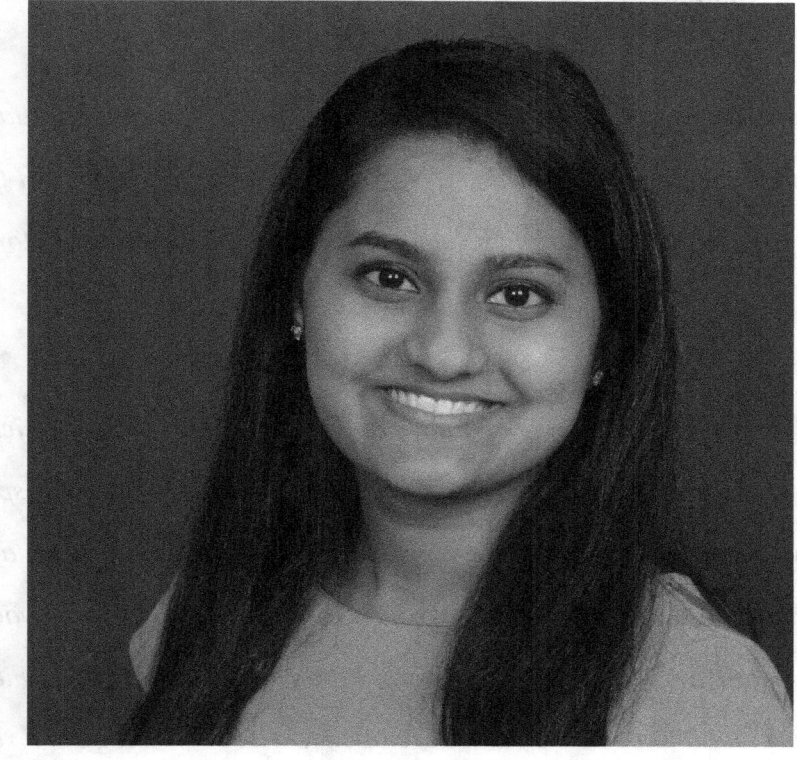

What were your experiences as an infectious diseases fellow during the pandemic? *We were assigned to run our own ID services as senior fellows. I was basically advanced to be an attending which was a completely new responsibility for me. It started with a lot of chaos. The entire hospital was looking to us for answers to COVID management, infection control, isolation, and screening questions. I had my own service of 10-15 patients and had 6-10 new consults every day. We were also in charge of the hotline to answer questions about how to do the nasal swab test and choose appropriate patient isolation. Initially we didn't have enough tests so we had to triage to see who would most benefit from testing.*

What factors did you use to triage which patients needed swabs initially? *If patients had respiratory distress, we asked them to come to the ER for oxygen therapy and further evaluation. If they were stable and without risk factors, we advised them to home quarantine.*

I had to rely on other providers' judgements over the phone, and I always erred on the side of being cautious and getting more testing done for patients.

How did things change as testing became more available? *Initially we had to reserve hospital testing for inpatients. If they were stable we did not test them on an inpatient and outpatient setting. As tests became more available, we could allow providers to make more of their own decisions.*

How does this pandemic compare to prior COVID-19 pandemics? *I think now there is a lot more travel and urbanization, the rate at how quickly the virus spread was much faster. Moreover, we have a lot more technology and resources these days to learn about the virus' genetic characteristics and have been able to start developing vaccines much faster. The communication of information across the globe is also faster which allows for the scientific information to be shared and developed faster. Technology and resources are on our side now compared to prior pandemics to start putting an end to this virus.*

What do we know right now about immunity to COVID-19? *There is a lot more known now than when the pandemic started. It would be strange for someone to have automatic immunity—it is a novel virus. If you have been infected and have antibodies, you are immune to the virus. I think a large percentage of the world is infected. I think that people who have not yet been exposed, can still contract the virus.*

For how long does immunity last? *With any infection, your body develops antibodies and memory cells to help fight the virus the next time you see it. You should be protected for life. When you get a vaccine, immunity usually lasts about a year to few years (depending on the type of virus). I don't really understand the scientific evidence about how we only have immunity to the virus for three months. It's not in line with what we know about immunology* *unless this is a new phenomenon which we may discover, but highly unlikely since time and time after we have studied how our bodies respond to multiple infections (viruses, bacteria, parasites and fungi)*

Why are herd immunity levels so low? We are testing IgG and IgM and there is definitely an antibody response to COVID. Herd immunity may be low because people are following proper precautions and so people are not being exposed. We are for the most part practicing a lot more masking and hand sanitizing overall which has reduced exposure. This definitely needs to be studied more and can change as our journey with this virus continues.

In 1918, most people who were infected in the first wave had immunity in the more lethal second wave. Do you think this could happen with COVID-19? If you had COVID in the past, you should expect some level of immunity to a mutated version and a less severe illness. Similar to the flu, where there are multiple strains, people who get the flu shot tend to have immunity to several different strains. Even if the vaccinated person receives a mutated version of the flu, we can expect a less severe infection. Of course this is a generalization and based on each case. I think the virus will mutate as it is an organism that is trying to survive in humans, but it is hard to accurately predict the future.

Are there any patient experiences that were particularly memorable to you? Most patients have had shortness of breath, chest x-ray changes with bilateral pneumonia findings—some more extensive than others. Sometimes you can see lobar changes that suggest superimposed bacterial infection. Not everyone needs oxygen or admission to the hospital. We are seeing endothelial damage and are seeing a lot of people with pulmonary embolisms. Now patients are started on anticoagulation to prevent this. In severe presentations, patients can have diffuse clotting, severe pneumonia, and multi-organ failure. Maintaining oxygen requirements was a big challenge. One other thing we saw is prolonged fevers. We tried to identify other *sources of infection, but more often than not it seems to be due to prolonged illness due to COVID. We have seen CRPs in the 40s which suggests a very severe immune response. A lot of time we try to re-evaluate why patients are still having fever and oxygen requirements to determine whether there is an additional source of infection or if these findings are due to inflammatory response. Usually it is the latter.*

What would you like people to know about COVID-19? *It is a challenging virus and we still don't know a lot. We should separate the economy and politics from the virus itself. There is scientific evidence on protective equipment not spreading COVID and healthcare facilities are trying to isolate patients properly. The news and media do tend to exaggerate things overall and sometimes are scientifically incorrect. We know how the virus spreads - from contact or droplets; aerosolized only in hospital procedures. There is a wide range of presentations for the illness and we are still learning about the virus, trying to gather the evidence we have day-by-day. I would say to keep up with scientific knowledge as much as possible. There is a possibility that a vaccine will be created in the near future, there is a lot of research and groundwork already done, we have come a long way in just a few months of a pandemic and I am excited to see what happens with this. I truly believe if we all work together, we are all collectively bigger than this virus.*

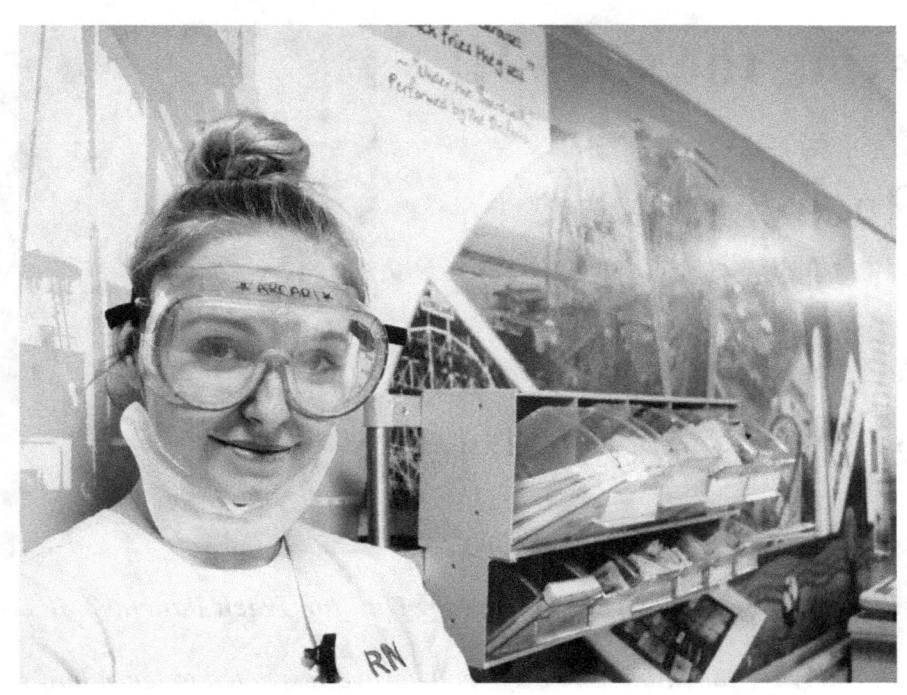

"This hospital is beyond amazing and has the best people you could ever ask to work with. I've never felt even close to alone on a shift. Everyone jumps in to help and always checks up on me knowing I'm a new nurse in this situation. This is a time where we're forming bonds with each other and growing as a team. The people I work with keep me motivated, inspired to perfect my craft, and make what should be an awful situation a positive experience every time I come to work."

-Audrey Arcari, Registered Nurse, Emergency Department Resident, NYC

Creating the COVID Recovery Unit

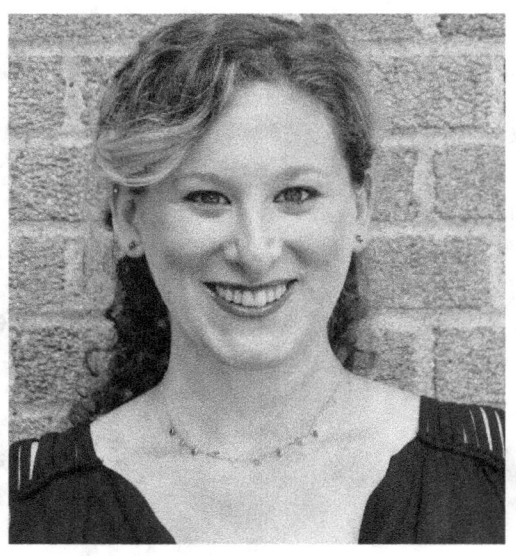

—*Dr. Kaile Eison, DO, Physical Medicine & Rehabilitation Resident Physician, NYC*

What was it like working at the COVID Recovery Unit for Trach Patients? *It's been incredible. Not really like anything I've ever done or ever expected to learn how to do. So much of it has been systems based—how to create a floor, work with other teams from other specialties, and to work with patients with unconventional rehab needs. The primary team on our trach unit is a military team with practitioners from emergency medicine, internal medicine, family medicine, and pediatrics. And we have our rehab team of PT, OT, SLP, social work—so we have been trying to collaborate to create a unit that serves the patients' needs.*

Can you describe your experience starting the COVID Recovery Unit? *That was intended to be a joint collaboration for medicine and rehab. We built a rehab floor with a gym and pulled in therapists from the acute side with the intention of creating a COVID positive space for patients to participate in rehab. Up until this point, COVID negative patients were allowed to go to the gym, but COVID positive patients had to stay in the room. We did struggle with a couple of things. Between the physiatry team and the hospitalist team, it was at times challenging to get everyone's expectations and needs met. Second, because it took* patients so long to get to that floor [due to high demand], a huge percentage of them were already swabbing negative soon after they got there. Although COVID negative, they were still unable to be transferred to an acute rehabilitation unit because they were so debilitated.

What kind of impairments do you see in the Recovery Units? Patients who come to the unit often have one or two comorbidities, not necessarily affecting them on a daily basis. But after prolonged hospitalization due to COVID, some of them have become so debilitated. These are people who are 40 or 50 days into their hospital course. We have a lot of critical illness myopathy and neuropathy, a lot of steroid myopathy, a ton of peripheral injuries—we suspect from proning. We see a lot of foot drop, brachial plexus injuries, and a lot of delirium. The cognitive impairments are really profound in this population. Oftentimes, even getting them to a point where they can participate in therapy takes a while, and the degree to which they can participate from a physical standpoint is very limited since they are so debilitated from having been in bed for so long.

What is the age of patients in the unit? It's a mix. I don't see a lot of the very old population—I think only a handful of those patients made it to rehab. I would say the majority are middle aged, 50s and 60s, and then we have a handful of much younger patients in their 30s who are equally impaired but who do recover quicker.

Minorities have been shown to be disproportionately affected by the disease. Do you see that in your units? There seems to be a much larger Hispanic population at both campuses *than we see in our typical acute rehabilitation units. At my hospital, approximately 70% of my patients are Spanish speaking only.*

You also got COVID. What were your symptoms like? *It was like a really bad cold. I was tested at one of the hospital testing tents. I had a stuffy nose, a headache, and 24-36 hours of myalgia and chills. It was a pretty quick recovery and I was ready to go back to work after a few days but had to stay out for the full 7 days.*

Your husband worked in ICU at one of the most severely affected hospitals very early in the pandemic. How did you feel when he was deployed there? *Early on it was very difficult. He would come home every single day and talk about so many of his patients dying and how they were out of ventilators and didn't have enough PPE. His job of having to pick which patients would get a ventilator, who would be able to be admitted—it was hard see him go through that and feel like I couldn't really help him. As patients started to recover and I was able to contribute more, in a purely selfish way it was a lot easier for me, because I felt like I was doing something productive! And now we have shifted. He is still seeing a lot of very sick people, but the COVID wave has crested over rehab at this point, so we are starting to get really sick patients.*

Are there any messages you would like to give to people about COVID-19? *It's so different going through it as a doctor and in New York than it is anywhere else, and it's so hard to convey that to people who are not here and not seeing it. I walk around and see people not wearing masks anymore or who are gathering in groups and I wish I could take them to work with me and show them what's it like for my patients who can't move and can't talk and can't* *think. It's such a multifaceted disease that affects every part of a person, and I don't think people realize that. It is still just a nebulous thing that people see or hear about in the news. It's a smell, and it's a feeling, and it's a tactile sensation being in the hospital with these patients and I wish I could convey that in a way to people who aren't there.*

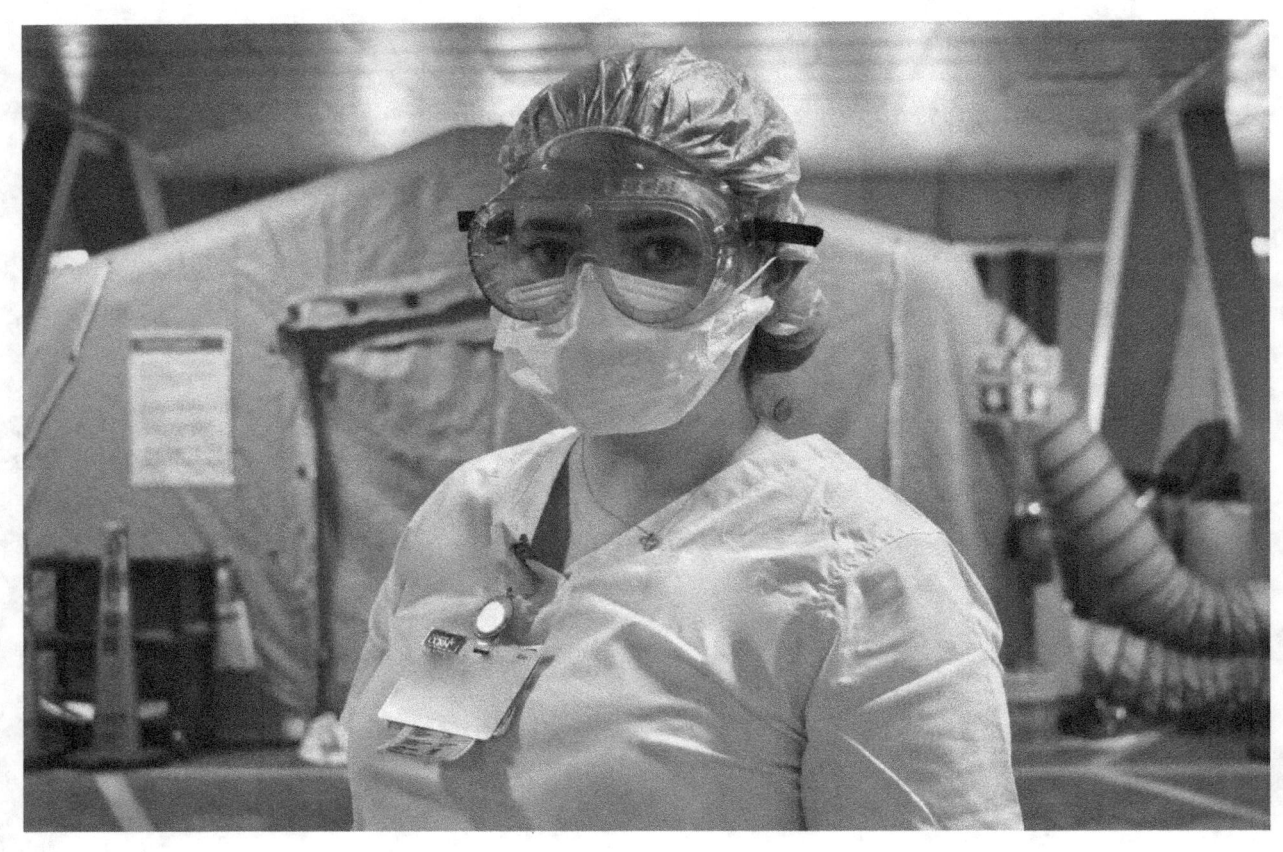

"We are NY Tough. This too shall pass."

-Katie Michels, Registered Nurse, Emergency Department, NYC

CHAPTER 19: WORLDWIDE IMPACT

"The final lesson of 1918, a simple one yet one most difficult to execute, is that...those in authority must retain the public's trust. The way to do that is to distort nothing, to put the best face on nothing, to try to manipulate no one. Lincoln said that first, and best. A leader must make whatever horror exists concrete. Only then will people be able to break it apart."

-John M. Barry, in *The Great Influenza*

On January 14th, the WHO declared the COVID-19 outbreak to be a global emergency. On March 12th, it was upgraded to a worldwide pandemic. In a mere 3 months, the disease has claimed the lives of over 400,000 people.

The following countries have reported more than 100,000 cases as of June 18th[46]:

Country	Reported cases	Deaths
U.S.	2,235,678	119,955
Brazil	960,309	46,665
Russia	561,091	7,660
India	368,705	12,280
UK	299,251	42,153
Spain	291,763	27,136

Peru	240,908	7,257
Italy	237,828	34,448
Chile	220,628	3,615
Iran	197,647	9,272
Germany	189,504	8,927
Turkey	182,727	4,861
Pakistan	160,118	3,093
Mexico	159,793	19,080
France	158,174	29,575
Saudi Arabia	145,991	1,139
Bangladesh	102,292	1,343

A complete review of the impact of COVID-19 in all countries would require a book to itself. The following is a brief overview of the impact of the coronavirus in several nations across the globe. Information about COVID-19 in China, Israel, India, Portugal, the UK, and South Africa, are discussed in other sections.

Australia

Melbourne, Australia, is one of the first major cities worldwide to reinstate strict lockdown after experiencing a spike in cases upon reopening. BBC highlighted residents' criticisms of stricter lockdown measures in poorer neighborhoods, where rates of infection have been higher, as compared to wealthier communities.

Brazil

The Brazilian president has criticized economic shutdowns, citing the fact that most cases of coronaviruses are mild. Brazil is the country with the second highest amount of cases. The indigenous population of Brazil has also gained press for its record number of deaths[85]. At greater risk due to their lack of infrastructure and access to healthcare, *CNN* reports that the community is dying at an alarming rate with a mortality rate of 12.6%-- double that of other Brazilians[85].

Bhutan

Bhutan has also had no COVID-19 deaths[44]. They helped orchestrate an 8,000-mile trip home for a 76-year-old American with COVID-19[44]. The patient survived[44].

United States

As of mid-June, America's death toll has surpassed 100,000 and we remain the most severely impacted nation, followed by Brazil. The United States was not as quick to lockdown as other countries, and studies suggest this may have contributed to the higher death rate.

India

India has the third highest death rate from COVID-19, but death rate remains relatively low in the second highest populated country. According to Anu Ganapathy, a resident of Bangalore, India initiated a strict lockdown early in the pandemic.

The United States has permitted four Indian companies to manufacture remdesivir and one is currently doing so. Nevertheless, reports of shortages of multiple medications abound. Remdesivir and toclizumab have been sold in the black market and significantly marker up pricing in New Delhi, India's capital city[49]. BBC reports that some families have spent their life savings to secure remdesivir, despite its limited clinical benefit in clinical trials[49].

The Taj Mahal re-opened for tourist visits on July 6th.[50] All tourists are expected to wear face masks and to refrain from touching the marbles surfaces[50]. Despite the reopening, tourist numbers will be limited to as low as 5,000 daily, as compared to the 80,000 daily tourists typically seen at peak season[50]. In actuality, even lower numbers are expected given continued strict lockdown measures in the communities surrounding the national monument.

Due to a surge of cases, the city of Bangalore will reinstate its lockdown from July 14th to 22nd. For my 81-year-old grandmother, the lockdown has been a disruption of her daily exercise routine and involvement with the community. She appreciates the government's measures to keep vulnerable people safe, including herself. The lockdown hasn't stopped her from exercising though—she still walks 1 hour daily on her terrace and performs 1.5 hours of yoga every morning.

Italy

In the early days of the pandemic in the United States, we watched in horror as the virus raged though Italy, resulting in over 230,000 cases and 33,000 deaths[104]. Why was Italy hit so hard? Italy has a high population of elderly citizens, with 22.6% of Italians over the age of 65 in 2018.[105] The country has a much higher population density than the United States, with 533 people per square mile as compared to 94 people per square mile in the U.S.[105] Rome has almost twice the population density of Washington D.C.[105] Northern Italy is also a business hub with close trade relations with China[105] As a result of these factors, Italian hospital systems were quickly overwhelmed and ventilators needed to be rationed. The U.S.

and other countries around the world were able to learn from the exponential and horrific rise of cases in Italy and instill preventative measures before experiencing such a surge in our country. Italy started to re-open in May, under pressure to do so from its economic devastation[44].

New Zealand

New Zealand has received considerable praise for its initiation of strict lockdown measures early in the pandemic, which is credited with keeping the number of cases very low. On June 8th, the country announced that it would end its strict lockdown as the country had no new cases[129].

South Africa

Like many other nations, South African is experiencing its worst economic recession in decades due to the COVID-19 pandemic[51]. Its budget deficit is expected to surge to 15.7%[51]. $2.6 billion of its $29 billion stimulus package will be allocated in October once its job-creation program and other projects have been further planned[51].

Sweden

As mentioned earlier, Sweden has been unique in its handling of the virus. Instead of quarantining its people, the Scandinavian country has released guidelines that more vulnerable members of the community self-quarantine and that others social distance and wear mask to limit the virus spread. The Swedish epidemiologist Anders Tegnell has advocated closing only aspects of society to help achieve herd immunity faster and prevent destruction of the Swedish economy. They have experienced a greater number of fatalities than neighboring Denmark and Switzerland. Tegnell continues to stand by Sweden's strategy, but relents that its greatest shortcoming was not providing greater protection to nursing homes where death rates have been highest[102].

Antibody tests have revealed 7.3% of Swedes were positive by Mid-May, though experts had estimated that the country would achieve rates of 40-60% by this time[125]. Again, I think that the lower antibody rates could be because those with mild or asymptomatic cases may be defeating the disease with a cellular response with antibody titers too low to be detected.

Despite its less stringent policy, the Swedish GDP is still expected to shrink 8% this year with an unemployment rate expected to rise to 10%[102]. In comparison, the U.S. unemployment rate is 14.7%[103], and the GDP of some other European nations is expected to shrink between 20-30%.

Vietnam

Vietnam has recorded no COVID-19 deaths[44]. "Patient 91," a 43-year-old British Airways pilot is in severe condition, requiring ECMO, a machine to help circulate blood to his lungs. Vietnam's health ministry has stated that the patient may require a lung transplant to survive, and Vietnam's government has spent $200,000 so far to search for a transplant from a clinically dead donor[44].

Lockdowns

In response to the virus, many countries have enforced lockdowns and curfews and declared states of emergency, crippling the global economy as 1.5 billion people are confined to their homes[30]. As a result of these measures, the global GDP is estimate to shrink an unprecedented 1% this year[30].

Slowly countries have started reopening. Greece has reported lower COVID-19 cases than many other European countries and is eager to restart tourism, which provides substantial income to its citizens[44]. Despite its low case rate, Athens is expected to have one of the worst pandemic-related recessions in the European Union[44]. On May 16th Greece started to reopen its beaches with strict social distancing rules and heavy fines for those who disregarded them[44]. Greece plans to reopen its restaurants and bars at the end of May[44].

On May 13th, the director of the WHO warned against prematurely opening lockdowns without widespread testing and community surveillance in place, stating "If the virus transmission accelerates and you don't have the systems to detect it, it will be days or weeks before you know something has gone wrong.

Countries such as India, South Korea, New Zealand, and Russia were expeditious and vigorous in their implementation of a lockdown and have been praised for their handling of the pandemic. India's case load pales compared to other countries despite its large and densely populated communities. My co-resident from Russia told me that when her father returned to Russia from travel abroad during the early days of the virus, he self-quarantined and law enforcement visited him daily and took his picture to confirm that he followed lockdown law! In a similar vein, a Russian man who took out his trash to the end of his driveway received a fine.

Some countries that reopened are now closing down again after a resurgence of infections. After a surge in cases during the Muslim holy month of Ramadan, Saudi Arabia will re-instate a total lockdown. In May, Wuhan, China, decided to test all citizens after a new coronavirus cluster has appeared, possibly from contact from infected arrivals from Russia[72]. Unnervingly, this cluster of cases shows a prolonged time to symptom onset as well as a prolonged recovery, suggesting that the virus could be mutating[72]. The delayed onset is also making it harder to catch the disease before it spreads[72]. Cases in the new cluster demonstrate primarily lung damage in contrast to the multi-organ damage seen in the patients of Wuhan and America[72]. Despite China's comprehensive virus detection system, it is still struggling to contain the new cluster[72].

With countries experiencing resurgences, there is the question of whether people can develop immunity to COVID-19. If not, can there be an end to social distancing if people can be re-infected? Until a vaccine is developed we are depending on herd immunity to keep vulnerable people safe. Not only are we still a long way from herd immunity, defined as 60% of the population, but if people can be re-infected the concept is moot.

Developing Nations

Developing nations will feel the brunt of both COVID-19 infections and lockdowns. We have seen across the world that populations that live in more crowded and less hygienic conditions and who have less access to healthcare are suffering from higher death rates. Furthermore, many of these countries have less capital to provide welfare for citizens in lockdown, increasing the risk of starvation and homelessness in those who can no longer work due to governmental restrictions. In the next chapter, I discuss neglected illnesses, and many of these are also more prevalent in developing nations.

Geopolitical Consequences

As wealthy nations witness economies collapse, what will happen if developing nations experience a surge of the virus? As the United States masses unprecedented amounts of debt, who will provide aid to countries in needs? Who will have first access to vaccines—countries who invest in their development or those who most need them? These questions loom as experts say a resurgence is likely, and it is unclear which countries will be hit hardest.

The WHO declares their goal is "to ensure that a billion more people have universal health coverage, to protect a billion more people from health emergencies, and to provide a further billion people with better health and well being[53]." Despite their tireless efforts to achieve and uphold this mission, the WHO has been criticized by its handling of the COVID-19 pandemic and President Trump is withholding U.S. contributions to the organization until a review is conducted[54]. Trump has stated that the WHO played a role in "severely mismanaging and covering up the spread of the coronavirus[54]…Had the WHO done its job to get medical experts into China to objectively assess the situation on the ground and to call out China's lack of transparency, the outbreak could have been contained at its source with very little death." America provides between $400 and $500 million annually to the WHO, ten times the contributions of China,[54] and Trump has discussed decreasing funds to the organization as well as the United Nations prior to the pandemic as well, stating that they were "ripping off" the United States[54]. In an interview with "Good Morning Orlando," Secretary of State Mike Pompeo said, "The World Health Organization in its history has done some good work. Unfortunately, here it didn't hit the top of its game." More than 100 countries have petitioned the World Health Assembly to conduct an unbiased review of the WHO's handling of the pandemic[28].

Let's Make Sure They're Comfortable

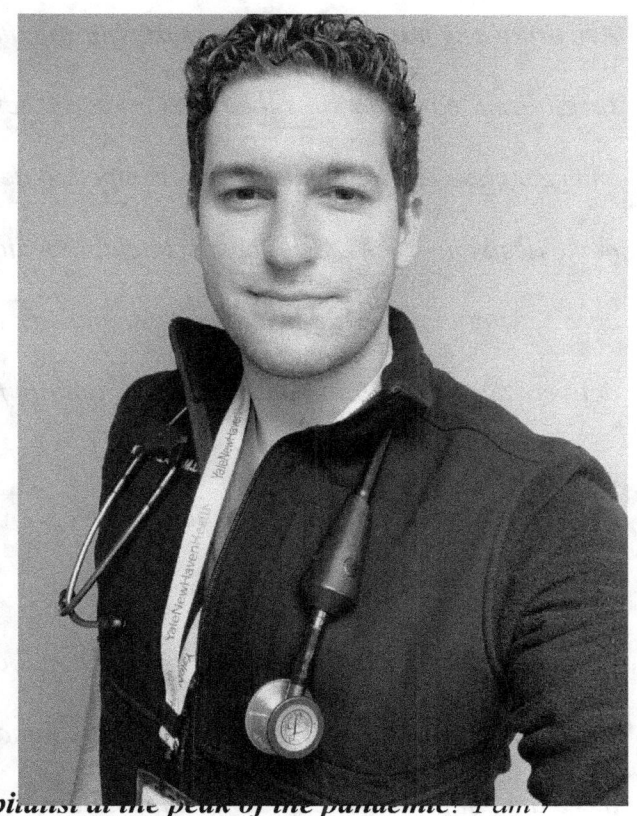

--Osama Kandalaft, MD,

Internal Medicine Hospitalist at

Yale New Haven Hospital, CT

What was your experience working as a hospitalist at the peak of the pandemic? *I am 7 months out of residency so am a relatively new attending. I have a lot less experience than my colleagues who have been in this field for much longer and have developed time-tested diagnostic and treatment algorithms based on the patterns they have seen throughout the years. But with COVID-19, we are all at ground zero. We have no experience with this disease and there is so much uncertainty.*

As a hospitalist, we work 12 hour shifts one week on, and one week off. After one or two days at home I start going crazy! I want to make sure I'm protecting the people I am caring for in the hospital by not going outside and bringing the disease back to them as an asymptomatic carrier.

Are there any patient experiences during the pandemic that most affected you? *We have a specialized team that runs the rapid response service and essentially handles all hospital emergencies. The team has been revamped to deal with decompensating COVID patients. We make decisions such as what experimental medications should be trialed and what level of care the patient needs. Most of our patients are elderly or with a lot of comorbidities, or actively decompensating and thus don't qualify for many treatments.*

I vividly remember being called into a case with a co-attending who was very seasoned. The patient was in her 50s and decompensating within hours of being admitted. She was initially on room air, then transitioned to nasal cannula, then nonrebreather. I entered the room and saw that she was barely breathing and non-responsive. My co-attending asked, "Is there anything else we can do for this patient?" I assessed the situation, similar to many I had seen before and pronounced, "No, I don't think there is any more we can do. Transition to comfort measures." Later my co-attending pulled me aside and asked how I stayed so calm during the decision and how I knew so readily and confidently that she should be CMO [comfort measures only]. And it hit me how we become so desensitized to the process, to the never-ending stream of COVID decompensations. We have become so used to saying "Let's make sure they're comfortable." It's not to say we don't care about these patients. We care about them deeply. There's guilt, stress, and regret when making these decisions. But ultimately, we know we are doing what is best for our patients.

What is it like for patients to not have visitors at the hospital? *I imagine myself at my most vulnerable when I am sick, my family can't come and see me whether they live a block away or in another country, and I don't have the capability to use the phone or communicate.*

Patients are isolated, which is insanely detrimental to their mental health and even disease progression. No one thinks to bring a phone charger when they are in medical distress and come into the emergency room. One of the best things I can do every day is to sit in my patients' rooms and interact with them. Essentially, we are the patients' providers, and we are also their family members.

What is it like treating patients with PPE? *You're putting on this medieval armor- the head gear, the masks, the shoe coverings, this mass of aprons. You're going into a patient's room and they can barely make out your eyes. You have 16-18 patients and you may have forgotten their names. It becomes very alien. You are no longer of their species. When patients see you, they are overcome with fear—how severe their disease must be if you have to gown up in all this every time you see them. The human touch is lost. Your visit is truncated in order to spend as little time in their room as needed, they feel a cold stethoscope on their backs, and then you're gone. Yale has identified this as a huge problem. Now, in every COVID positive room they have a computer screen with a camera that you can pop on any time to see your patients and chat with them. Unfortunately, due to security concerns, family members are unable to use these devices. Staff often use their own phones to facilitate video chats with family members.*

What do you want people to know about COVID-19? *Just be open about what you see and what you read. I'm not talking about studies from NCBI or bulletins from the CBC. I'm referring to the conspiracy theories.*

There's also the idea of selflessness. People are losing jobs, can't see their family members, can't take vacation, and are being told to stay home. I think it's easy to fall into the routine of individualism where we think about "me". I want to go out, I want to get a haircut, I want to get a beer with my friends. I urge people to think about the community and the people. It's not us who are suffering. Whatever the stress and strain and the lack of resources, you're harming your neighbor if you don't social distance or don't wear a mask. Our focus and obsession with the individual may need to take a breather to save our community.

Final thoughts? *We're in a real-time episode of House that's not ending. We just don't know so much about this disease- how it works, why are certain people at so much higher risk for severe disease, is my treatment hurting you or making things better?*

We are seeing an unprecedented support for all types of healthcare. I was walking to work the other day and there was a tiny sign that said "Thank you healthcare workers. Stick in there." Just seeing that was enough to keep me going another 3-4 days. It's an acceptance by society that we are trying to do the best that we can. That appreciation helps us endure the 12 hour shifts on our feet, transcends our fears and uncertainties.

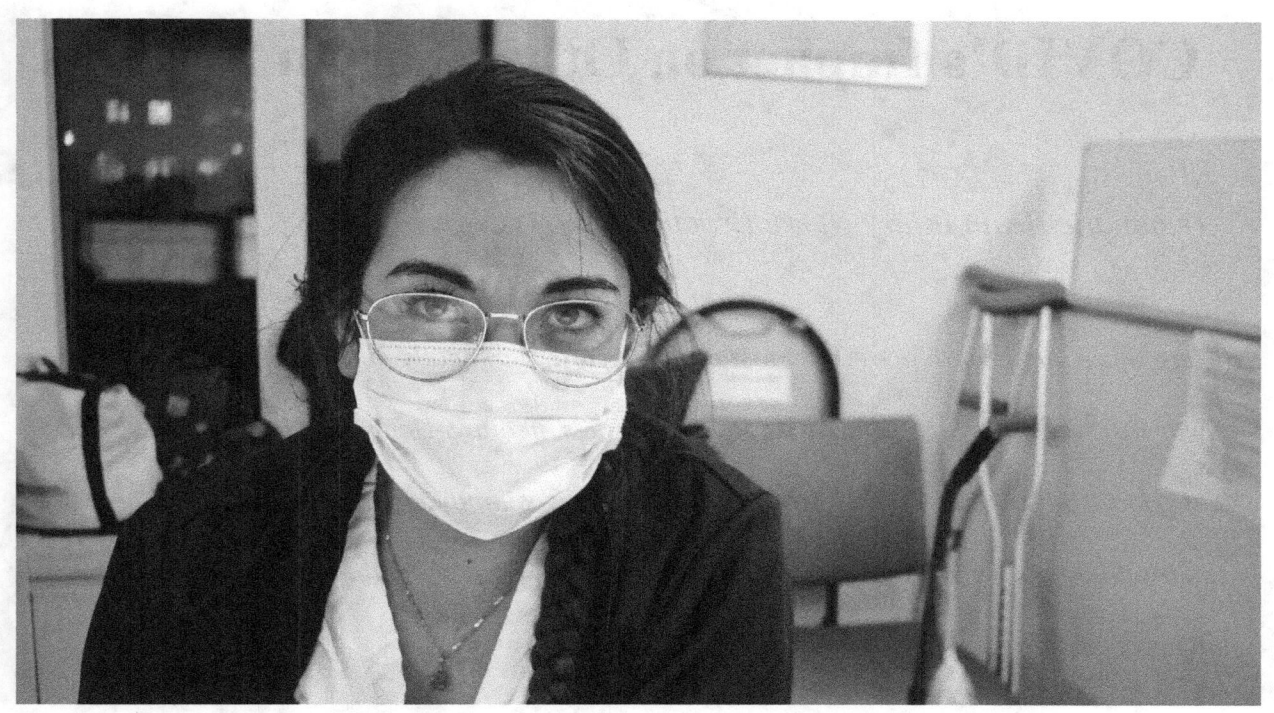

"One of the hardest things is trying to reassure my family that is outside of NYC that I'm okay, I'm being safe, and we are doing our best. I'm lucky that they are a bit removed from the hot zone, and that I have people who are worried for me. But it's hard to reassure them with words. I wish they could see the way our hospital has come together as a team through all of this. It's amazing. I love what I do, and the fact that I am with my friends through all of this is such a privilege. I couldn't do this without them."

- **Samantha Jewell, Registered Nurse, Emergency Department, NYC**

COVID's Impact on Other Organ Systems

-Traumatic Brain Injury Nurse Practitioner, NYC

Were there any experiences that most affected you? *Personally, my friend's husband passed away last week. He was 53, no other medical issues, healthy. He used to exercise daily and eat good food. He had COVID 4 weeks ago and he was intubated. He had a cardiac arrest post-intubation. We went to school together and she has young children—one is graduating this year and one is 13.*

Fortunately, I was able to decannulate [remove the trachs] all my COVID+ tracheostomy patients, and they were able to go home. Even patients with severe encephalopathy were able to go home.

How has working during the pandemic impacted your family? *My family in India are healthy. They were very scared for me and called me regularly. They wanted to make sure I was taking care of myself. My family in Kuwait is getting the full course of COVID right now. Thankfully, my family is safe but it is crazy over there. Now when I go home I change my scrubs, my shoes, take a shower. I don't want to bring the virus home to my in-laws, who are older and with co-morbidities.*

What would you like people to know about COVID-19? *I have had patients who tested COVID negative but they were jaundiced [their skin was yellow] and had significantly elevated liver enzymes. I don't think the nasopharyngeal swab is reliable in these patients. We* *may be seeing later effects of their disease course. We are all concentrating on the respiratory part, and there will be more to learn regarding its effects on the liver, the kidney, the GI system, the blood system. Maybe we will need fecal testing. We are still not completely aware of the full course of the disease and there are a lot of things we have to learn.*

Author's Note: I am this last point was brought up. Just this week I presented a journal club article on how COVID positive patients continued to have positive fecal testing after their respiratory swabs were no longer negative. The authors conclude that fecal testing may be necessary to prevent fecal-oral spread. I have discussed with my attendings the possibility that COVID+ patients may continue to be spreading the virus through fecal transmission even once they test negative on nasopharyngeal testing. This is of especially significant concern in our spinal cord and traumatic brain injury patients, who require extensive daily bowel regimens to prevent severe constipation.

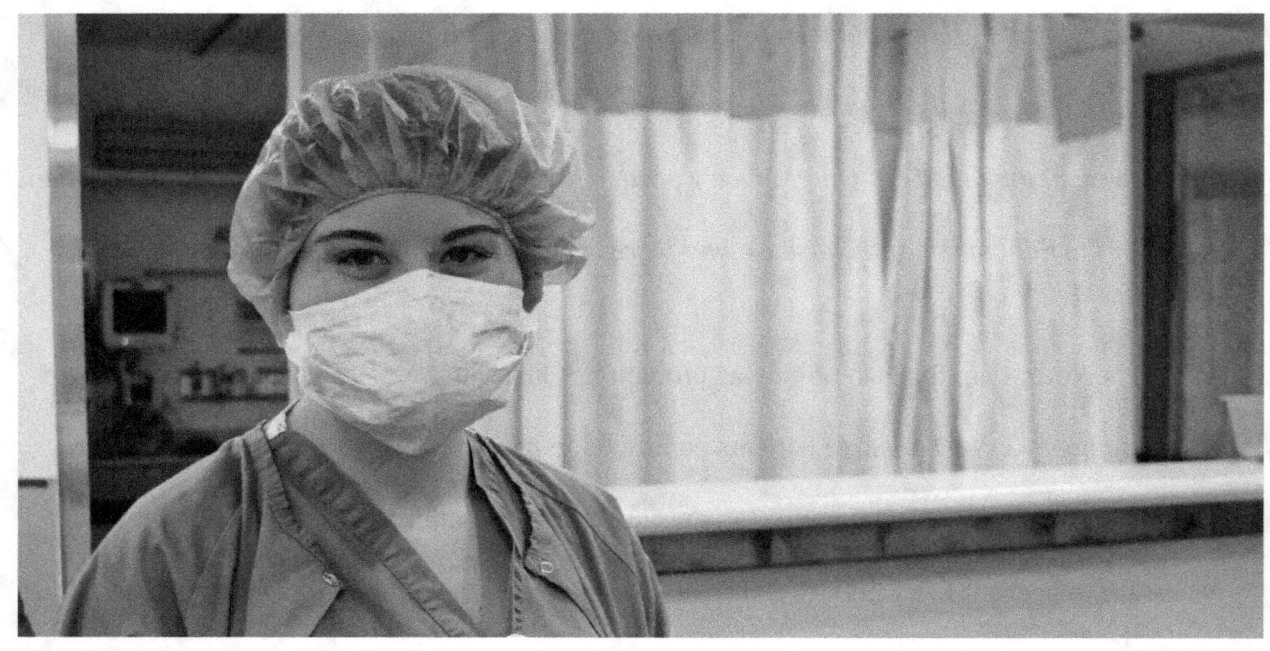

"I am so happy that I am able to come over and help out during this tough time. It is inspiring to see nurses from all different hospitals and departments working together as one to treat these patients and fight the pandemic."

-Kaitlyn Kelly, Registered Nurse floated to the Emergency Department, NYC

CHAPTER 20: NEGLECT OF OTHER ILLNESSES

"The COVID-19 pandemic is like nothing we have seen in our lifetimes. We must do everything possible to lessen its potential destructiveness. Part of that is also making sure we do not forget about the other important care patients require to stay healthy and function. If we do, we risk emerging from this crisis with a population and workforce much less able to contribute in making our societies and economy strong again."

-Timothy Hoff, PhD, Professor of Management, Healthcare Systems, and Health Policy at Northeastern University in Boston, MA[111].

Elective surgeries and procedures and in-person primary care appointments have been postponed. Some people feared seeking needed care at risk of exposing themselves to COVID-19. Others were unable to receive care due to revised hospital policies and government regulations. What will this postponement in healthcare mean for baseline physical and mental health? Worldwide, as resources have been relegated to COVID-19, they have been drained from fighting other serious global illnesses, and implications may be far-reaching and long-lasting.

Tuberculosis (TB) support groups in India have expressed fear that they will have a 4.5 million increase in TB cases over the years since many of their patients have been unable to seek care due to quarantine. The WHO and UNAIDS have estimated that a 6-month interruption in antiviral therapy for AIDS could result in 500,000 more deaths due to the AIDS in Sub-Saharan Africa in the next two years[28]. The disrupted treatments are because HIV services have closed, the supply chain has been interrupted, or because services are now overwhelmed with supporting the response to COVID-19[29]. Furthermore, mother to child transmission of HIV is expected to increase by 104%[29]. Says director-general of the WHO Dr. Tedros Adhanom Ghebreyesus, "The terrible prospect of half a million more people in Africa dying of AIDS-related illnesses is like stepping back in history."

The WHO and UNICEF have warned that as vaccination rates decline and other illnesses are neglected, there has been a surge of vaccine preventable infections around the world. Diphtheria has increased in several countries and a mutated strain of poliovirus has spread through more than 30 countries[119]. Cases of measles, much more highly infectious than COVID-19, have exploded in 18 countries, and the ensuing measles epidemic could kill more children than the coronavirus[119]. MMR vaccine rates have also dipped in the United States—with a 63% decrease for all children and a 91% decreased for children over age 2.

The UK has reported a 700% increase in calls regarding domestic violence[31] and it is possible that levels of depression will increase as the economy deteriorates, leading to increased mental illness and decreased quality of life.

A *New York Times* article questions "Where are the other patients?" because of the sharp decline in stroke and cardiac ED and hospital admissions during the pandemic. Patients with chest pain who would otherwise have called 911 may be afraid to go to the hospital lest they be infected with the coronavirus, thus foregoing care. The U.K's National Health Service released data that shows urgent cancer care referrals have fallen by 60%[120]. It is estimated that an additional 18,000 people will die of cancer in the U.K over the next year due to COVID-related disruptions in treatment, including missed diagnoses due to a decrease in screening, and fewer cancer surgeries, chemotherapy treatments, and radiotherapy sessions[120]. This number approaches 40,000 in the United States[120]. How much morbidity and mortality may be caused *as a result of* COVID-19 lockdown, fear, and supply-chain disruption?

Fady Asly, the Executive Chairman of the International Chamber of Commerce in Gerogia, made a striking comparison of deaths from COVID-19 to deaths from other conditions, based on Worldometer data. From January 1 to May 14 of 2020, here is a list of the most common causes of death around the world:

Abortions: 15,663, 274

Cancer: 3,025,690

Smoking: 1,841,683

Alcohol: 921,423

HIV/AIDS: 619,313

Road traffic accidents: 497,318

Suicides: 395, 065

Malaria: 361, 364

COVID-19: 290,000

Influenza: 179,336

Fady also states that epidemiological simulations estimate that at least 50% of any population will ultimately be infected whether or not a lock down is in place[30]. The National Institutes of Health says that obesity and overweight together are the second leading cause of preventable death in the United States, causing an estimated 300,000 deaths per year[55]. Heart disease kills 1 person in the United States every 37 seconds resulting in 647,000 American deaths annually[56].

The lockdown has served its purpose in preventing the overwhelming of our healthcare system, and thus prevented needless deaths due to a lack of ventilators, hospital beds, and healthcare providers. At the same time, it has devastated the world economy and may result in a greater number of deaths from untreated TB, AIDS, heart attacks, strokes, depression, suicide, poverty, and food insecurity.

Food for thought…Why has the world been shut down for COVID-19 when the number of deaths from abortions, cancer, smoking, alcohol, HIV/AIDS, road traffic accidents, suicides, and malaria all out-number COVID cases, and we still allow driving, smoking, and alcohol use? The world has mounted a monumental response to COVID-19. Why not against these other preventable conditions that result in so much more death and morbidity on a daily basis? Why is obesity—a reversible condition that triples the odds of severe symptoms from

COVID-19—not treated as a public health emergency? As the global GDP continues to shrink, unemployment rates surge, and the global poor bears the burden of economic shutdown, policies that save life *and* quality of life need to be considered.

New Nurse in the ICU

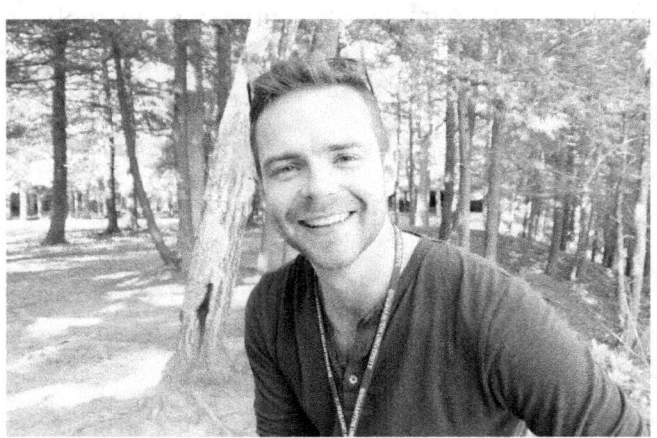

—*Julien Deshler, RN, ICU Nurse, NYC*

What was it like to be a new nurse in the ICU at the peak of the pandemic? *I am a very new ICU nurse. I enjoy ICU nursing, but starting here during the pandemic has been challenging.*

I had COVID at the end of February. I treated my first COVID patient and 5 days later I spiked a fever. I was wearing proper PPE so I'm leaning more towards it being community acquired. When I came back, my unit was entirely COVID positive. Everyone was vented and very sick with this mysterious virus. I remember seeing all our IV pumps outside the rooms. This was, for obvious reasons, quite overwhelming. Not only were we concerned about the well-being of our patients, but our own mortality was at the front of our minds. I am lucky enough to work for an institution with centuries of history that has built political connections and has quite a large reach. Thankfully, the staffing and PPE was never as limited as at some other city hospitals. Overall, the experience was challenging, but I felt very supported. In terms of skills and device practice, I got lots of experience with ventilators, and continuous renal replacement therapy... more so than I probably would have otherwise on orientation. That was probably the only upside to the whole situation though. On my worst day, I had 3 COVID vented, critically ill patients, some requiring CRRT [Continuous Renal Replacement Therapies].

Were there any patient experiences that particularly affected you? *A lot of critically ill patients required dialysis and ended up being trached. Thankfully, many recovered their renal function and were able to clear drug metabolites that were keeping them sedated. Now in May, we are finally discharging people that were admitted in March. To see an active functional member of society suddenly become critically ill, vented, sedated, and on the edge of dying is heartbreaking. But we have had more success than we expected. People are getting better. Although the road to recovery will be long for many.*

Did you see many patients die from COVID-19? *We have seen a lot of patients pass away. At the beginning of March, we had several deaths per day and it was really hard for everyone.*

Did you see any interventions that benefited ***patients?***

Normally, once patients reached us they were severely hypoxic and intubation was imminent, or had already occurred. But we did have a patient we were able to hold off from intubating for an extra 4-5 days by awake proning. We were using hydroxychloroquine for a while but did not see obvious or significant benefits. This is a rudimentary and biased observation though, just a disclaimer. I've given remdesivir to a couple of patients. In those with mild to moderate disease it may help, but by the time patients reach us, they were already 2-3 weeks into their disease process and seem to have progressed into a different disease phase more characterized by a hyper immune response. I'd be curious to see if steroids could help blunt this response and save lives. Another disclaimer: there is no research on this at the time and this is purely based off intuition.

Is there anything you would like people to know about COVID-19? *It's a reminder to all of us to make the best of the time we have with the people that are important to us. It has been challenging for a lot of people to unexpectedly not be able to see their loved ones for months, or forever if they passed. I've heard families say, "I really wish I had said [this]", or "I wish I had more time with [him/her]." Try to make the most of the time that you have with your loved ones. Use this quarantine opportunity or others in the future to be reminded of the transient nature of our experiences with others.*

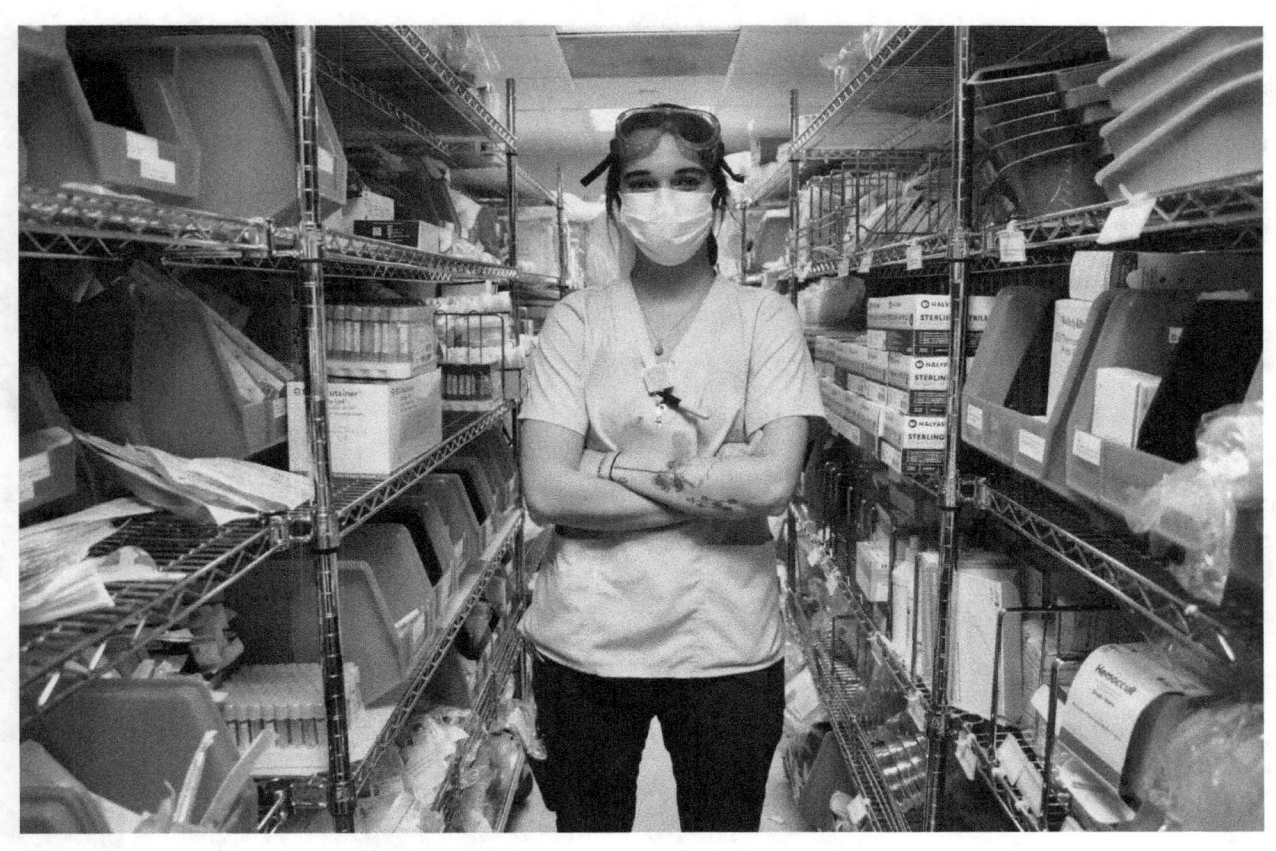

"I could never even put into words how much I admire and appreciate my coworkers. They've truly been there on my best and worst days and I know will continue to be there every day until we overcome this pandemic. I'm hopeful that people will listen. This is VERY REAL and it's not going away anytime soon unless every single person is on the same page and STAYS HOME. We CAN do this."

-Abigail Moss, Registered Nurse, Emergency Department, NYC

On the Proning Team

- Lance DeGuzman, Occupational Therapist, NYC

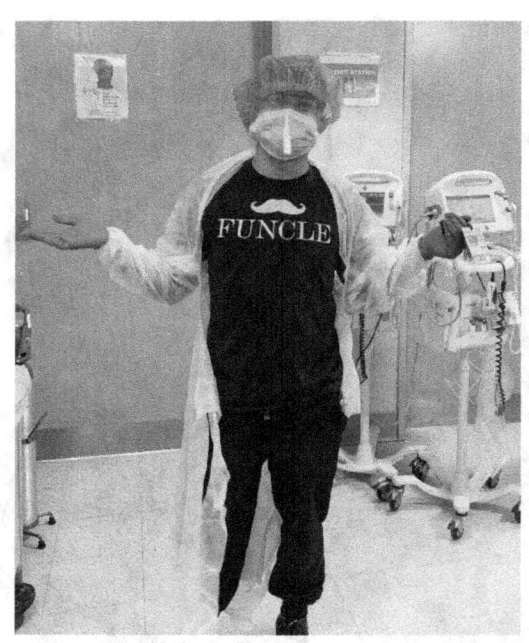

How has the pandemic affected your life? *It has taken away a lot of my meaningful outlets (such as traveling and family time). I actually missed the birth of my nephew which is the reason behind the photo above. I used to see my family every single weekend but have been unable to during the pandemic. Now as things have eased up we have found a good middle ground of seeing each other while remaining socially distant!*

What was it like to care for COVID-19 patients at the peak of the pandemic? *It feels like a blur. There was immense fear in the beginning. But we answered the call because these patients needed us. Now it has become the new normal. We know that after a traumatic experience, things become a blur, and all of us have experienced that with this virus. I was part of the proning team. I worked with a lot of the patients who were knocking on death's door.*

What was it like to be part of the proning team? *Therapy has never been involved with proning before. We knew what it was but no one did it because it was usually in the nursing arena. We shifted to longer working hours, our caseload tripled, and we did back to back proning or supine sessions for multiple hours straight. When I reflect back, our focus was on proning as many patients as possible, and we never got a second to really see patients for who they were, which is a large part of our usual therapy.*

Have you returned to traditional occupational therapy as COVID cases have decreased?

Prone team is done and we are back to occupational therapy, but nearly all my patients are recovering from COVID. There is SO much deconditioning, pressure sores, brachial plexus injuries. I also get to work with patients who were proned during their hospital stay. It is very rewarding to see the progression of their recovery.

Final thoughts?

There's a video of Cardi B talking about coronavirus. She says something like "It's real and it's coming and the Bitch is scared." I feel like that sums it up pretty well. It is sink or swim and we swum in order to do the best for our patients.

Author's Note: When looking up the exact Cardi B quote, I read that Cardi B has donated $1 million to struggling families amongst the COVID-19 pandemic, along with 20,000 meal supplement drinks to NYC medical professionals. Way to go Cardi B! I also shared with Lance that most providers I have spoken with say proning in addition to oxygen therapy was the most helpful intervention in treating COVID-19 patients. Thank you, Lance, and your proning teams for your tireless care that saved many lives.

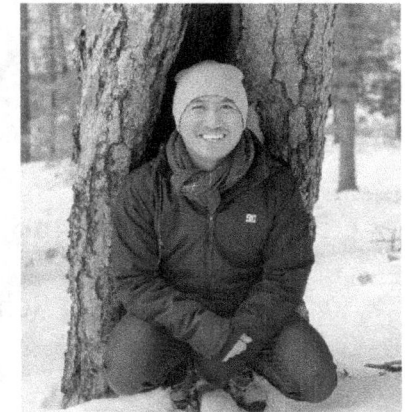

CHAPTER 21: RESURGENCE

"It is likely that any relaxation will lead to some resurgence. The goal would be to have the resurgence be monitored and contained. So you relax guidelines for some people first, do extensive testing to watch for a resurgence and then, if all goes well, you can relax guidelines for others. Priorities for who should have their restrictions relaxed first will need to be determined at the local level with a lot of different stakeholders included in those decisions. The populations that are identified as high risk of severe disease would likely be last to have their restrictions relaxed."

-Ryan Malosh, PhD, Assistant Research Scientist at the University of Michigan School of Public Health

Dr. Fauci and other health experts have stated that a resurgence will be inevitable. Analysis of prior pandemics reveals that it is common for there to multiple "waves" of novel viruses due to new outbreaks or mutations. In the 1918 pandemic, the second wave of the pandemic was much more lethal than the first[101].

From mid-June to early July, as all states have begun reopening, there has been an expected increase in cases. States that were spared early in the pandemic have understandably had the highest spikes in cases. The University of Washington estimates that at an additional 80,000 Americans will die from COVID by November[128].

Planning for Resurgence

Most physicians I have spoken with agree that hospitals will be better prepared for a resurgence than we were for the initial onslaught. We have protocols in place now, and the ability to amass ventilators, PPE, and ICU space if needed. The importance of maintaining flexibility, such as the ability to redeploy our workforce and to convert beds to ICU level of care, will be crucial. Hospitals and health care providers who have trained in different specialties need to have intensive care experience to meet the demand if needed once again.

> **If I am infected in the first wave of COVID-19, will I be spared in the second?**
>
> In the 1918 pandemic, the majority of those who were infected in the first wave of the disease were spared in the more lethal second wave. This is likely because their bodies were able to recognize the similarities in the second strain of the virus and mount a monumental immune response to stop viral replication early in disease course. Though we can't know for sure, it is possible that those who have already been infected may be immune or have less severe symptoms in a second wave.

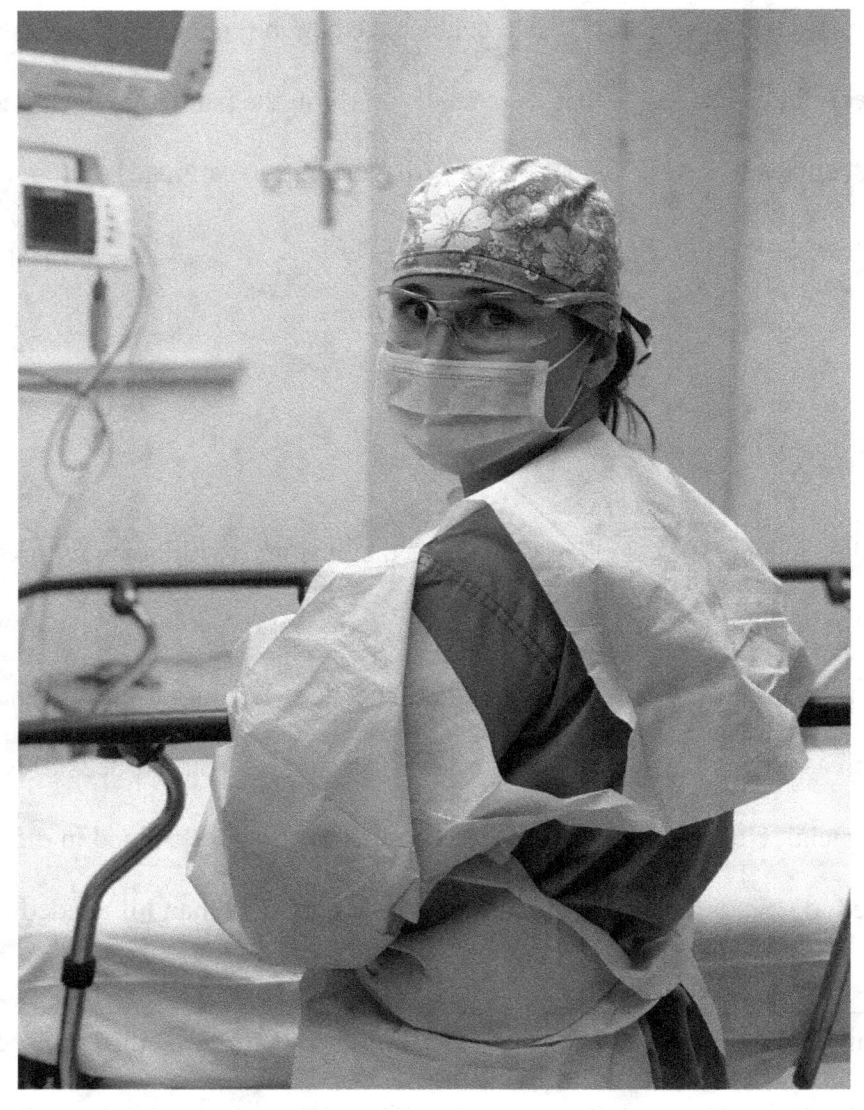

"Albeit a lonely, scary, and sad season, I have never felt surer of my decision to be here. It is times like these, when we are called on to be where it is hard to be, that I feel most unwaveringly sure that I want to be here. Going on months of battling this virus, we are being tested in a new way. We keep getting up to do it again, not knowing

when or where the light at the end of the tunnel may be. As we are tested in this way, endurance, grit, grace, creativity, and presence to one another becomes more important than ever. The fact that this is hard does not always need to be sugar coated with silver linings. Sometimes joy can be a little more all-encompassing, and can look a little more like a sleepy NY nurse watching movies with her dad in Boston via Facetime. We can be sad for the world AND grateful for silver linings AND lonely AND happy to see tulips AND restless for this to be over. Maybe that can be joy too."

-Adelene Egan, Registered Nurse, Emergency Department, NYC

Reflections from the COVID Service

-Dr. Ritu Nahar, MD, Internal Medicine Resident Physician, PA

"Be inspired by fantasy but coordinate it with reality. Tranquility and honest reflection will reveal passing illusions"

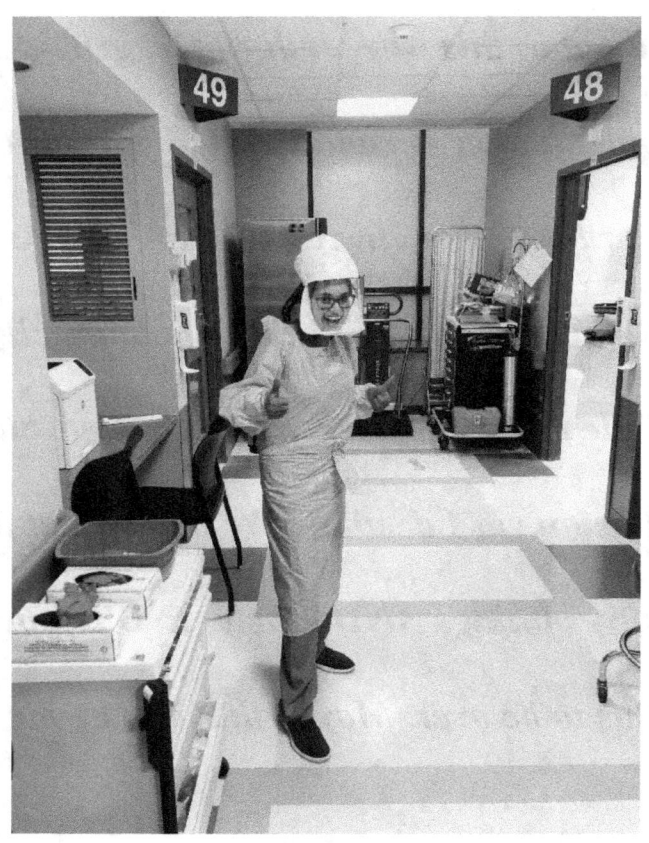

Prior to starting the Covid service, I was eating and drinking fear and anxiety- there were wakeless nights and internet research, scrutinizing countless emails taking notes on the latest Jefferson Covid guidelines. I was altering between feeling like a strong and resilient knight in the face of this mysterious ferocious virus to an imposter knight cowardly fearing the impending doom while basking in the existing gloom. Upon starting the service, the anxiety within the hospital was physically and psychologically palpable. As the routine of being on the Covid service began to normalize I quickly realized there was actually little we could offer patients. I now dug for the courage to face my sense of powerlessness as I admitted repeatedly to patients and their family how little we could offer. I felt like I was on a palliative care rotation my first week, just making everyone DNR/DNI watching them perish on

nonrebreathers. But there were those that made it! The couple that persevered. The 90-year-old sassy Haitian lady who still drove her daughter home from the Bronx, where she worked as a nurse (also Covid +). But there were days that broke me. I remember the fatigue as I consciously chose not to go visit Mr. P's wife/family when they came to say their final goodbyes.

I'd read the news and feel rage towards those not following the social distancing protocols. I felt betrayed by the government who chose to ignore warnings of scientists for which our nation now stood woefully unprepared against this pandemic. Because even after I left the hospital, I couldn't escape it. The virus was a silent stalker. It could be on my shoes, on my clothes, in my hair. Even as I took precautions stripping down at the door, showering what felt like an inordinate number of times I felt isolated and consumed by the unknown risk I carried of getting this goddamn virus or carrying it asymptomatically. I felt isolated from my family, from my boyfriend, and my roommate. This was a pretty significant disruption to my social support and there was no defined end date.

And I am now off the service, still feeling fatigued and anxious. I know I am an anxious person. This has been a lifelong struggle. But I reflect on my weeks and find myself saying "it wasn't even that bad!" I had an awesome team (that Bollywood video still makes me smile!) I was able to do my part. I feel healthy. Why the fuck do I feel so uneasy. Maybe because I start the ICU with Covid + patients again? Maybe it's my selfish anxiety. After seeing what could and has happened to my patients and family friends. The implications of what could happen to my direct family. My friend's dad passed of a sudden MI, Covid +. My family member is in the ICU on ECMO, Covid +. My mom is going to the hospital scoping Covid + patients. My grandparents are in India, is this lockdown doing to be enough to protect them all?

I had been trying to cope by just being indifferent. By trying to keep busy. But that is a facade, as my underlying anxiety slowly leeches my energy while I attempt to rejuvenate in my face masks listening to Alt-J. They say no one will protect your suffering. I'm hoping writing this out will allow me to acknowledge the impact this experience has had and is having on me. I'm accepting this experience is pretty fucking shitty and the impact is magnitudes far beyond me. But I think in the midst of all this I am allowing my anxiety of the morbid possibilities, of the things I can't control, squelch my ability to stay connected with myself/others and maintain a sense of inner peace. It's like Nature was observing our society from afar and now has made her presence known, bringing us to our knees making us question- what really matters to you? I can choose to indulge in my anxiety or just surrender to the suffering this has and will cause while doing my part. When I ask myself how I will I go on, I'm reminded of this quote from Sheryl Strayed:

"You go on by doing the best you can. You go on by being generous. You go on by being true. You go on by offering comfort to others who can't go on. You go on by allowing the unbearable days to pass and allowing the

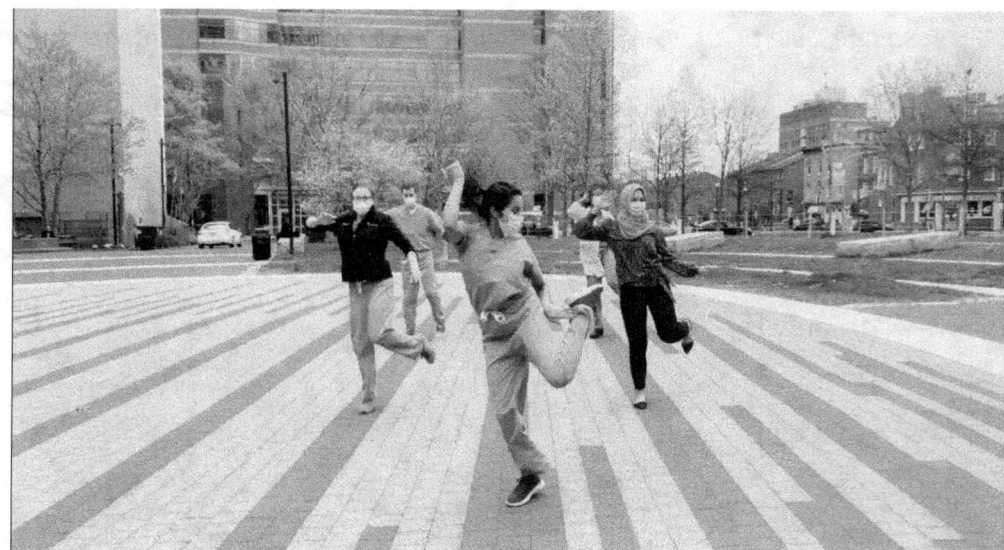

pleasure in other days. You go on by finding a channel for your love and another for your rage."

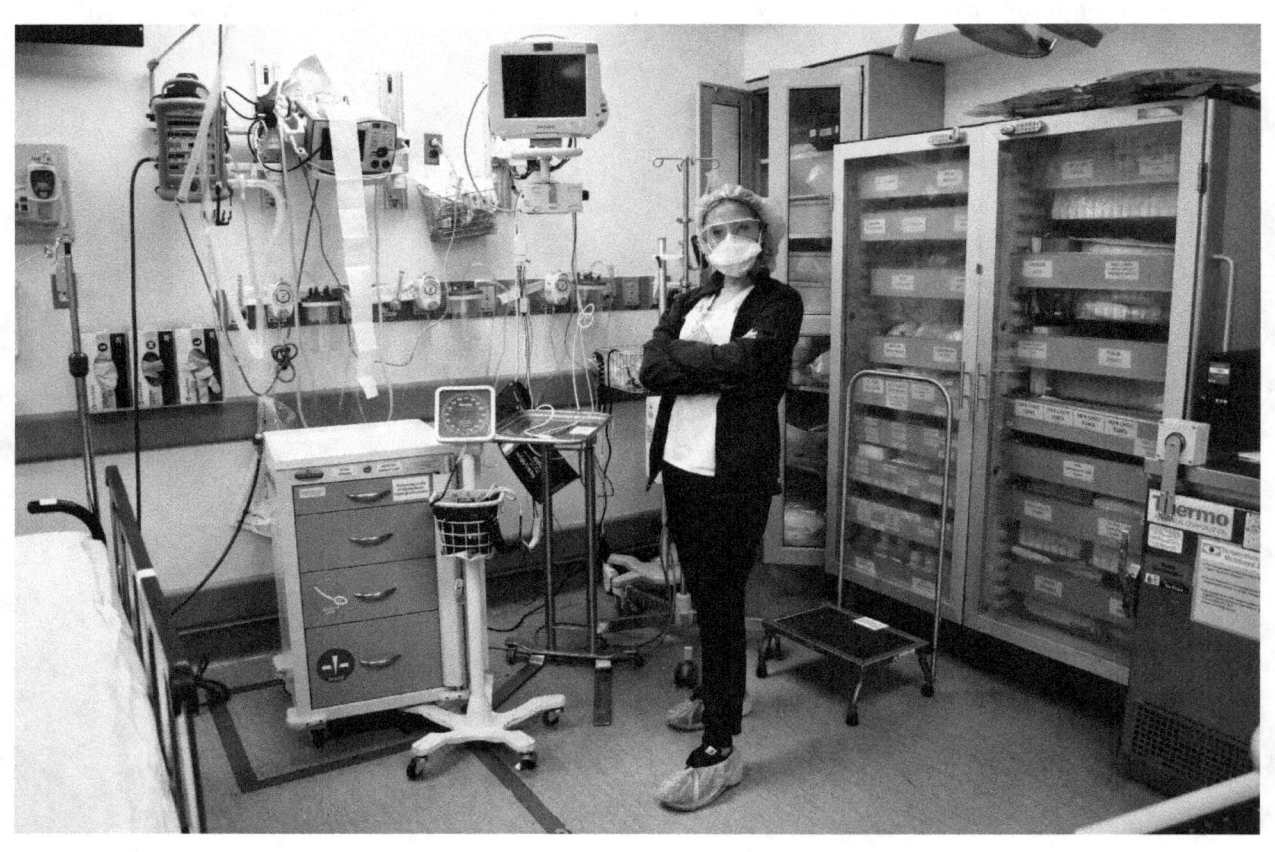

"Being on the frontlines of the pandemic has created some uncertainties and fear but it has not changed the way I view my career. I have always shown up to work ready to be the best nurse I can be with hopes of bringing a little positivity to people during their darkest days. Nothing about that has changed. I hope in the weeks, months, and years to come that people still remember to be supportive and kind to healthcare workers. We are always trying our best. My coworkers have been my rocks through this crisis. They are

always there when I am in need of help or a good vent session. They are calm, kind, and supportive. I truly have the best team by my side every single shift!"

-Chloe Bowman, Registered Nurse, Emergency Department, NYC

Letter from Dr. Michael Prodromou, MD, Pulmonary Critical Care/ICU Attending Redeployed to Mt. Sinai Queens, NYC

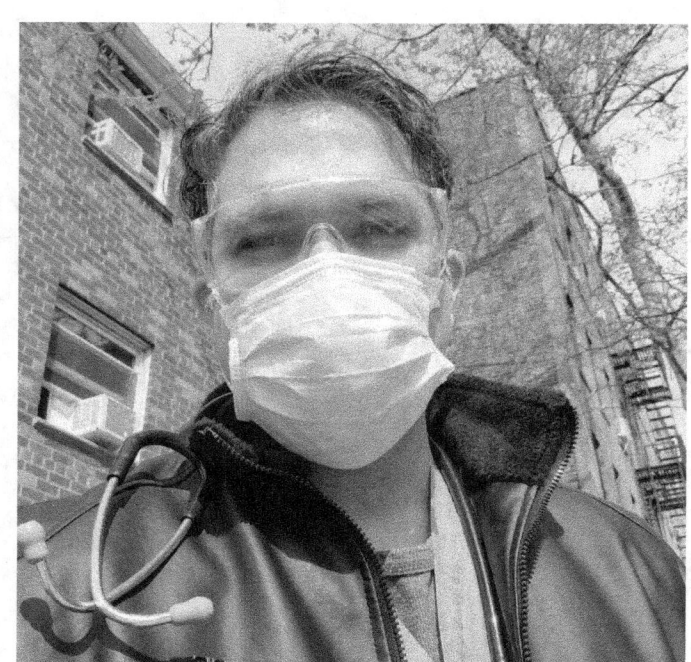

May 24th:

This is a few days late as I needed time to collect my thoughts. This past week marked the end of my redeployment to help in the fight against COVID, and since then I have been moved back to my home base at Mount Sinai Doctors of Long Island outpatient pulmonary clinic.

It was a tough 6 weeks. I spent all my free time in isolation, away from my wife and family, as I was too concerned about unknowingly infecting a loved one. All of my interactions with people outside of the hospital were in the form of telephone calls, texts or video chats. I spent a lot of time Lysoling and Cloroxing things that I never cleaned before – amongst them my car steering wheel, face shield, and the floors of my apartment, all as part of a lengthy daily decontamination process that once upon a time would have been perceived as obsessive compulsive but now seems to be a norm for those on the frontlines.

The first few weeks were the toughest as we struggled to meet the demand of the patient load and to adjust to the new normal. The ER and floors were full. Many didn't make it. It felt at times like we were in a warzone. Over time, however, things became more routine. Our knowledge about this disease and how to treat it improved. We celebrated small victories - a discharge here, a ventilator liberation there. "Here Comes the Sun" would be played over the speaker system every time a patient was discharged - it was always the same snippet of the song. Part of me wonders what I'll feel when I hear the song again in the future. Pride? Anxiety? Will it transport me, even for a brief second, back to April 2020?

I always wanted to be a physician ever since my younger years. When a child tells you that they want to "help people," you know that their ambitions are coming from a good place. The road to get there, however, can leave even the purest dreamer disillusioned. So you want to be a doctor? Great! Just take AP courses in high school, rock the SAT, get a 4.0 and do a bunch of research in college, crush the MCAT, make yourself stand out amongst all the other stand outs in medical school, keep doing research, smile and nod every time a resident/fellow/attending decides to go on a power trip at your expense, spend your best years doing overnights and 70+ hour work weeks so eventually you can get the attending position of your dreams in order to meet your RVU goals, research publication requirements, argue with insurance companies and all the while don't forget to look out for your liability. Don't get me wrong - I'm not complaining, and I wouldn't change my job for anything in the world. That was not 100% my experience, but you get the point. The road to becoming a doctor is rough. Being a doctor, though rewarding in so many ways, is not easy.

During my redeployment, for the first time, I felt unencumbered by all the roadblocks that I dealt with on a daily basis. Everything just melted away. In the hospital, it was just me, the patients, my peers, the virus, and nothing else. I was fulfilling that raw, unfettered dream of helping people, and I was doing it with the bravest, most selfless group of doctors, nurses, pharmacists and respiratory therapists assembled, some of whom came from all over the country just to help out. In the beginning, the idea of going to a COVID hospital in the epicenter of the outbreak was intimidating. Then, I saw the amazing comradery amongst all the healthcare workers and the enormous potential to make a difference for those who were in their greatest time of need. Never before had I been so proud to be part of the healthcare community. After getting used to a new normal and developing a routine to stay safe and decontaminate, it wasn't as scary. In fact, the hospital became my safe place.

The COVID hospital is the safe place? How could that be? In the hospital, there are infectious diseases, but we can control them. PPE. Washing hands. Being smart. It's not that difficult. Outside the hospital, there are many other infectious diseases – this includes COVID, but also hysteria, fear mongering, conspiracy theories, temptations to break social distancing guidelines, and political finger pointing. Unfortunately, there is no PPE for these types of diseases.

I'm not sure when the transition occurred, but the outside world became more anxiety provoking than going to the hospital or COVID itself. When you try to run an errand, get to the store and see a large crowd, many without masks, all of a sudden, the hospital feels safer than public areas. Couple that with endless news sources spinning the story of COVID to fit their agenda, Facebook posts arguing one way or the other, widespread anger, finger pointing and distrust, and it becomes apparent that the real warzone is not the hospital, but the reality that we contest amongst ourselves.

"China is to blame. Wet markets. The virus was created. Trump's fault. Obama's fault. Fauci's good. No Fauci's bad. Plandemic. Cuomo for president. No, he's working with Gates. Stop funding Blue States. Shoot up Lysol. Fund Boeing. I need a haircut. Stimulus check. Big Pharma's plan to make money off of us by selling us a cure. Liberate this, liberate that. The media is the virus. 100,000 deaths."

It's tiring to endure all of that day in day out. I'm not sure how people so fervently believe the opinions brought forth on social media, and how they all of a sudden developed an urgency to fight a social injustice against fill in the blank - big pharma, vaccines, the government, Trump, Biden - now in the middle of a pandemic, at the potential harm of loved ones.

So, with this post, as something different, I offer you thanks. Thank you to all my friends and family who texted, messaged me or called me to check in on how I was doing. Thank you to all the teachers in my life that helped me get to this point. Thank you to all my peers that taught me so much along the journey. Thank you to everybody at Brown – residents, fellows, attendings, nurses, that helped shape the doctor I am today. Thank you healthcare workers and all types of essential workers that risk their lives every day. Thank you to all of you that had to endure sacrifices because of shelter in place. Thank you to all those that I had worked with during my redeployment.

I'm glad that things are getting better. As much as I would love to upload a photo giving you a thumbs up and captioning it, "Mission Accomplished," we are not completely in the clear. Even though we are about to reopen, that does not mean that we can drop our guard. Complacency breeds failure. Let's do this safely and responsibly.

I can't say that I'm thankful for this experience, because like each of you, I would rather have not had to go through it. However, because of this experience, I got to help people on a level that I never was able to before. I learned a lot about my own personal fears and limitations, but I also learned about my strengths. I am more thankful for all my friends and family and for working alongside other doctors, RTs, nurses, MAs who are the living embodiment of diamonds being formed under pressure. I hope when the sun finally does come, we will be able to greet it stronger and more united than ever.

It was the honor of a lifetime.

FINAL MESSAGES

On May 26th, I am ready to deliver another journal club presentation. This time the presentation is via Skype and the topic is COVID-19 in spinal cord injury patients. We are in the process of writing a case series of our six COVID positive spinal cord injury patients, to share our knowledge in treating the disease in this vulnerable population.

I think back to the journal club I delivered two and a half months earlier and reflect how the world has turned upside down during this time. There are over 8 million people infected with COVID-19 and more than 400,000 deaths. The global economy is devastated. And yet we are on the uptrend. The number of cases at our hospital decreases every day. The U.S. economy has been showing early signs of recovery as the country re-opens. Our people continue to be hopeful and indomitable.

Despite the sadness, fear, financial and emotional turmoil caused by the battle, it has been inspiring and humbling to see our community band together to fight this virus. The love, support, and appreciation has been palpable and provides the fuel and energy for essential workers to continue this battle. Free meals for hospital workers, food delivered to our vulnerable community members, parents simultaneously working from home and teaching their children—COVID-19 has changed our way of life but we will defeat it. TOGETHER.

I hope this book helped answer some of your questions regarding the novel coronavirus, and inspired you with the experiences of our frontline heroes. If you have any further questions or comments, I would love to hear from you. Please write to me at krutika_parasar@alumni.brown.edu to continue the conversation.

Best wishes, Krutika Parasar Raulkar

Book Group Discussion Questions

1) Do you have any personal or professional experiences from the pandemic that you would like to share with the group?

2) What are your thoughts regarding the medical response to COVID-19?

3) What are your thoughts regarding the government response to COVID-19?

4) Which of the healthcare provider interviews/reflections in this book most affected you and why?

5) What strategies have you used to stay mentally strong during the pandemic?

6) If you are a parent or student, what were your experiences with remote learning?

7) Would you take a vaccine when it becomes available? Why or why not?

8) What do you think about the many illnesses that are being neglected as a result of the global lockdown? Can you think of a solution to this problem?

9) What do you will be long-term impacts of the pandemic on people and society?

10) If you have any personal experiences you would like to share, if you would like to send a message to any other healthcare providers in this book, if you would like to obtain a discounted bulk purchase order, or if you would like to donate to the family of Priya Jose and others who have lost a loved one to COVID-19, please feel free to email me at krutika_parasar@alumni.brown.edu.

Recommended Reading

These are books on pandemics that I read myself prior the COVID-19 pandemic. They are excellent reads and I highly recommend both!

The Great Influenza: The Story of the Deadliest Plague in History by John Barry

Amazon Synopsis:

Magisterial in its breadth of perspective and depth of research, *The Great Influenza* provides us with a precise and sobering model as we confront the epidemics looming on our own horizon. As Barry concludes, "The final lesson of 1918, a simple one yet one most difficult to execute, is that...those in authority must retain the public's trust. The way to do that is to distort nothing, to put the best face on nothing, to try to manipulate no one. Lincoln said that first, and best. A leader must make whatever horror exists concrete. Only then will people be able to break it apart."

At the height of World War I, history's most lethal influenza virus erupted in an army camp in Kansas, moved east with American troops, then exploded, killing as many as 100 million people worldwide. It killed more people in twenty-four months than AIDS killed in twenty-four years, more in a year than the Black Death killed in a century. But this was not the Middle Ages, and 1918 marked the first collision of science and epidemic disease.

The Plague by Alfred Camus

Amazon Synopsis:

A haunting tale of human resilience and hope in the face of unrelieved horror, Albert Camus' iconic novel about an epidemic ravaging the people of a North African coastal town is a classic of twentieth-century literature.

The townspeople of Oran are in the grip of a deadly plague, which condemns its victims to a swift and horrifying death. Fear, isolation and claustrophobia follow as they are forced into quarantine. Each person responds in their own way to the lethal disease: some resign themselves to fate, some seek blame, and a few, like Dr. Rieux, resist the terror.

An immediate triumph when it was published in 1947, *The Plague* is in part an allegory of France's suffering under the Nazi occupation, and a timeless story of bravery and determination against the precariousness of human existence.

Acknowledgements

This effort was a group collaboration by so many willing, engaged, and enthusiastic health care providers and community members. I am so thankful for the contributions of my colleagues and friends, and for the continuous referrals I received to expand the breadth of experiences in this book.

Let me start at the beginning, with my family—my lifelong support in everything I do. Thank you to my Patti, my grandmother who lives in Bangalore, India, for being the first person to read this book. You taught me to read when I was in preschool and have fostered my love for reading ever since. Thank you to my mama, my editor, for reviewing countless additions of the book and always believing in my writing ability. Thank you to my father, for realizing that medicine was the right fit for me before I did, and always encouraging me to aim for the best. Thank you to my husband for believing in this book and urging me to publish it fast while it was relevant, rather than waiting for a traditional publisher. I have learned about the field of independent publishing because of you and I love it! To my brother for your comments and for referring me to Bhu Srinivasan for advice regarding the publishing process. Thank you for also sharing your experiences with ScoreTrade. To my in-laws Ai and Baba for your love and care for me, Ajinkya, and Riaan and Risa. Though I put you at risk by bringing COVID-19 home to you, you have always been so supportive of my work. We couldn't have made it through the pandemic without you. To my wonderful aunt and uncle, Anu and Sanjay, who have been a lifelong source of love and support. Anu, thank you so much for referring me to many of your friends around the world—Danny Naidoo, Yatish Garach, Pukka Pajamo, and Nandini. I was amazed at how quickly you all responded to my requests for interview and it was enriching to learn about your experiences in other countries. To my children, Riaan and Risa for being my pride and joy and my greatest source of happiness.

To my NYP family…Thank you Vera Tselina, for your cheerful demeanor, infectious laugh, and constant desire to learn, it has been such a pleasure to work with you this year. Thank you Kaile Eison, you were my first interviewee and your eloquence and passion inspired me to do many more. Thank you, Dr. Rosenberg, for all your teaching and kindness during my residency. I am in admiration of your calm and patience when covering multiple services. Thank you to Dr. Stein—we are all so appreciative to have you as our chair. We admire your approachability, kindness, and knowledge of the field. Thank you to my program director Dr. Visco for your weekly updates during the pandemic and your support throughout residency. I have rarely seen you without a smile on your face and I appreciate how much you care you for your residents and patients. Thank you to Camille Culbengan, Emily Jackson, Laura Riley, and Ansel Oommen for allowing me to share your *HealthMatters* excerpts. Thank you to to the team at *HealthtMatters* for kindly letting me share their excerpts. To Lorenzo and Lance, thank you for your expert care of our rehabilitation patients and your cheery attitudes. It is always wonderful to speak with you and I am so happy you shared your experiences in this book.

My Stamford colleagues…Stamford Hospital was a wonderful place to train and provided me with my foundation in medicine in an inviting and comfortable environment…Thank you to Theodora Vamvouris, one of my dearest friends from intern year, for contributing and referring so many colleagues to me to share their stories! Thank you to Dr. Babayev, our renal attending, for responding immediately with my request to interview her for this book. And thank you to Dr. Streett, for all your teaching during my training and for taking the time to share your experiences as an infectious diseases expert.

Mt Sinai…Thank you to Anthony DeVivo and Michael Prodromou for interviewing with me, and to Mike for also sharing your Facebook posts. Your posts reached many during the peak of the pandemic and were vital in sharing healthcare providers' experiences with the community, and I am so thankful you readily allowed me to include them in this book.

Public Relations/Administration/Human Resources/Compliance…Thank you to Dr. Laura Wasson, Mrs. Wallaine Walters, Mrs. Maureen O'Shea, Mr. Chuck Mazer, Mrs. Terry Puchley, Dr. Christine Lauren at NYP; Robert Hutchinson at Yale, Adam Dvorin at University Hospital, Sinthuja Vigneswaran at Mt Sinai, and Stamford Hospital Media Relations for taking the time to my book and ensure compliance.

Thank you to my neighbor Susan. Our hour-long hallway conversation inspired this book. It is amazing how social interactions inspire creativity, and I am thankful to have had you as a kind and caring neighbor these past three years.

Thank you to Jessica Faust at BookEnds for being the first agent to respond to my book. I am so thankful for your advice to include the physician experience, which transformed my book.

Thank you to NYC Council Member Andy Cohen for your daily updates regarding the medical and service related COVID-19 news. They were a wealth of information to me, and I'm sure, the rest of our community during these challenging times.

To my contributors…Dr. Craig Smith, thank you for permitting me use of your updates in this book, although they ultimately did not make it in. They are so beautifully written and an excellent capture of the hospital's response to the pandemic and I think they will be a great asset to the pandemic literature when published one day. To Adelene Egan who responded with utmost enthusiasm when I asked her to join this project. Your photography is beautiful and you have helped to recognize so many brave healthcare providers who provided crucial care during the fight against COVID-19. Thank you to the ED staff at Cornell who responded with encouragement, praise, and enthusiasm to be involved when I asked to include your photos and quotes.

To John M. Barry, I so admire your book *The Great Influenza,* and it greatly inspired me to write this book. Thank you for allowing me to quote your work, for your supportive correspondence. It was wonderful to learn that you are a fellow Brunonian!

Thank you to my extended family Jyothi and Anju for interviewing with me and sharing your experiences, and for your love since I was born. You are like second mothers to me and I was thrilled to be able to collaborate with you on this book. Thank you to Devyani for your masterful editing, you are like a sister to me and your contribution meant so much.

Thank you to Jessica Faust at BookEnds for being the first agent to respond to my book. I am so thankful for your advice to include the physician experience, which transformed my book.

Thank you to NYC Council Member Andy Cohen for your daily updates regarding the medical and service related COVID-19 news. They were a wealth of information to me, and I'm sure, the rest of our community during these challenging times.

To Priya and your sons, thank you for sharing your painful memories regarding your beloved husband and father. You are so brave and so positive, and I think of your family every day.

To Megan for sharing my message with your friends and colleagues and referring me to Catherine Migel. Thank you, Catherine, for sharing your personal and professional experiences! Thank you to Lorna Hopkinson, Diane Fox, and Cristina Cianci (CC) for putting me in touch with your friends and family who had experiences to share.

To all my loving friends and family for supporting this book, and for your texts and concern for me during the pandemic. You mean so much to me and I hope you enjoyed this book. Special mention to Surina Diddi, who took the time to review and edit the book—so thankful for your time and help and life-long support!!

To all the essential workers who risked their own health to care for their communities during the pandemic. You are all heroes and we are thankful for your sacrifice.

About the Author

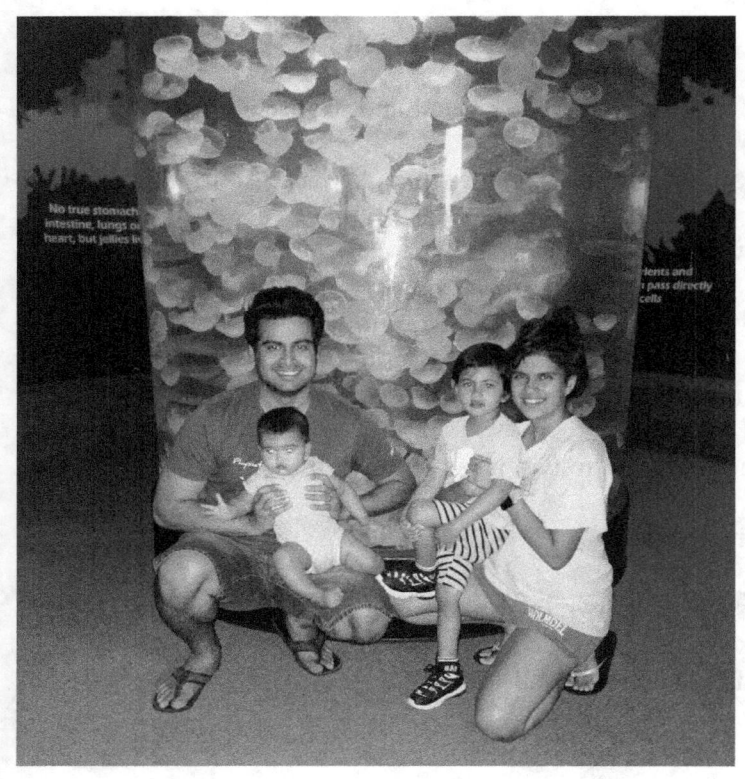

Krutika Parasar Raulkar completed her Physical Medicine and Rehabilitation residency at NewYork-Presbyterian Columbia/Cornell, where she served during the pandemic. She graduated magna cum laude from Brown University in 2012 and attended Rutgers Robert Wood Johnson Medical School, where she was elected to the Gold Humanism Honor Society and received distinctions in Medical Education and Community Service. An exercise enthusiast, she has run three marathons and enjoys a myriad of sports/fitness activities. Her first book, *Exercise as Medicine,* was published by *Wild Brilliance Press* in 2018. The same year, Dr. Raulkar was featured on the Dr. Oz show for her care of Montel

Williams after he suffered a stroke and received rehabilitation at Weill Cornell Medical Center.

Following residency, Dr. Raulkar moved to Chapel Hill, North Carolina, where she lives with her husband and children—her lifelong partners in health and happiness.

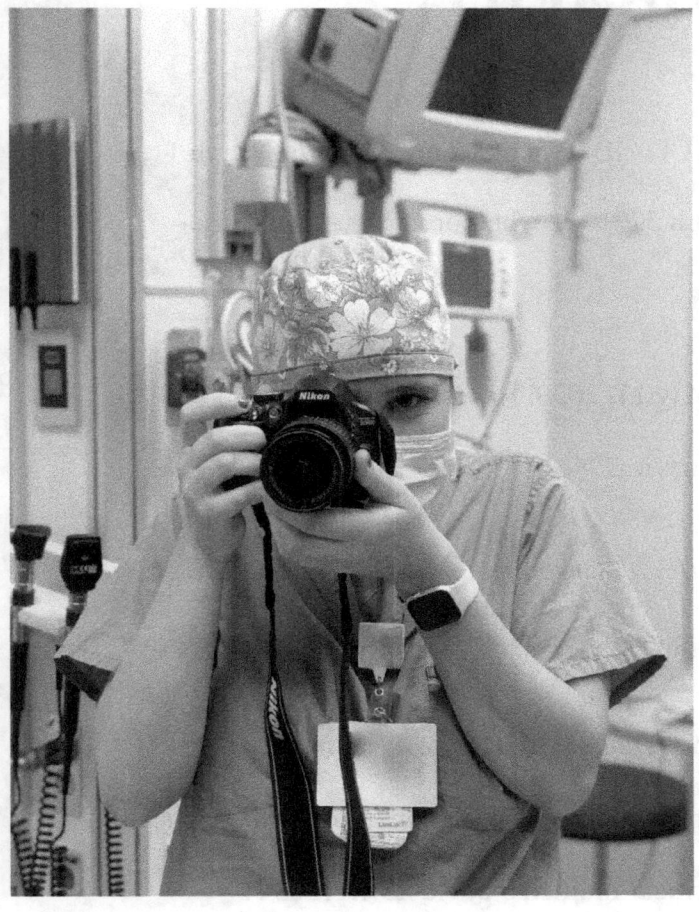

About the Photographer

Adelene Egan is a Boston native turned NYC Emergency Room Nurse who has pursued photography as a hobby for the last several years. She earned her bachelors in nursing from Boston College during which time she completed a semester abroad in Manila Philippines, partook in a number of missions in Jamaica and Ecuador, and volunteered with Boston's Healthcare for the

Homeless program. Outside of being a nurse, Addie enjoys traveling, hiking, and spending time with her friends. Addie is currently pursuing a Masters in nursing education with the vision of mentoring and supporting new nurses as they grow into the holistic caregivers, advocates, and resources that patients need. At the center of her practice as a nurse, Addie's goal is to care for people in mind, body, and spirit. Addie continues to fight COVID at NYP Cornell in Manhattan, and is ready for whatever may come because she feels upholstered by the love of her city, family, and friends.

BIBLIOGRAPHY:

1) "World Health Organization Declares COVID-19 a pandemic." *TIME*. March 11, 2020. Accessed from < https://time.com/5791661/who-coronavirus-pandemic-declaration/>

2) "Coronavirus Cases." *Worldometer*. May 11, 2020. Accessed from <https://www.worldometers.info/coronavirus/>

3) "WHO Timeline COVID-19." *World Health Organization*. April 27, 2020. Accessed from < https://www.who.int/news-room/detail/27-04-2020-who-timeline---covid-19>

4) Muccari, R et al. "Coronavirus timeline: Tracking the Critical Moments of COVID-19." *News*. May 22, 2020. Accessed from < https://www.nbcnews.com/health/health-news/coronavirus-timeline-tracking-critical-moments-covid-19-n1154341>

5) Stolberg, SG. "Fauci Plans to Use Hearing to Warn of 'Needless Suffering and Death.'" *The New York Times*. May 11, 2020. Accessed from <

https://www.nytimes.com/2020/05/12/us/politics/coronavirus-fauci-senate-testimony.html>

6) "Preliminary In-Season 2019-2020 Burden Estimates." *CDC*. Accessed from < https://www.cdc.gov/flu/about/burden/preliminary-in-season-estimates.htm>

7) "Coronaviruses." *NIH: NIAID*. Accessed from < https://www.niaid.nih.gov/diseases-conditions/coronaviruses>

8) Ghinai, I et al. "First Known Person-to-Person Transmission of Server Acute Respiratory Distress Syndrome." *The Lancet*. March 13, 2020. Accessed from < https://pubmed.ncbi.nlm.nih.gov/32178768/>

9) Duarte F. "Who is 'patient zero' in the coronavirus outbreak?" *BBC*. February 24, 2020.

10) Zhe, Xu (2020, February). Pathological findings of COVID-19 associated with acute respiratory distress syndrome. *The Lancet Respiratory Medicine*. 8 (4): 420-22

11) Adult Tracheostomy Placement and Care. *New York Presbyterian Hospital*. May 12, 2020.

12) Hannah. "Say Goodbye to These Stores That Are Closing Shop This Year." *Beach Raider*. March 18, 2020. Accessed from <https://www.beachraider.com/worldwide/off-st-ta/5>

13) "ACE-2: The Receptor for SARS-CoV-2." *R&D Systems*. Accessed from < https://www.rndsystems.com/resources/articles/ace-2-sars-receptor-identified>

14) Yang Y et al. "The deadly coronaviruses: The 2003 SARS pandemic and the 2020 novel coronavirus epidemic in China." *Journal of Autoimmunity*. May 2020. Volume 109. Accessed from<https://www.sciencedirect.com/science/article/pii/S0896841120300470?via%3Dihub>

15) Gu, J. and C. Korteweg (2007) Am. J. Pathol. **170**:1136.

16) Schoeman, D. and B.C. Fielding (2019) Virol. J. **16**:69.

17) Fehr, A.R. and S. Perlman (2015) Methods Mol. Biol. **1282**:1.

18) Centers for Disease Control and Prevention. *Common Human Coronaviruses*. Accessed from <https://www.cdc.gov/coronavirus/general-information.html>

19) Lu, R. *et al.* (2020) Lancet. **395**:565.

20) Zhou, P. et al. (2020) Nature [Epub ahead of print].

21) Hoffmann, M. *et al.* (2020) Cell [Epub ahead of print].

22) The Washington Post (May 13, 2020). Live updates; colleges opening in the fall is up for debate; grave alarm raised for economy.

23) The Washington Post (May 13, 2020). California state university, the nation's largest 4-year system.

24) ARUP Laboratories (April 21, 2020). How Accurate are Coronavirus Tests? Many Factors Can Affect Sensitivity, Specificity of Test Results

25) Zou L, Ruan F, Huang M, et al. SARS-CoV-2 Viral Load in Upper Respiratory Specimens of Infected Patients. *N Engl J Med*. 2020;382(12):1177–1179. doi:10.1056/NEJMc2001737. PMID: 32074444

26) Wu LP, Wang NC, Chang YH, et al. Duration of antibody responses after severe acute respiratory syndrome. *Emerg Infect Dis*. 2007;13(10):1562–1564. doi:10.3201/eid1310.070576

27) Wu F, Wang A, Wang Q, et al. Neutralizing antibody responses to SARS-CoV-2 in a COVID-19 recovered patient cohort and their implications. medRxiv. [Epub ahead of print].

28) Ravelo JL & Jerving S. COVID-19: A Timeline of the Coronavirus Outbreak. Devex. April 29, 2020.

29) World Health Organization. The Cost of Inaction: COVID-19 Related Service Disruptions Could Cause Hundreds of Thousands of Extra Deaths from HIV. May 11, 2020.

30) Asly, Fady. A Few of Us May Die From COVID-19, But the Current Lockdown Will Kill Many More People. March 26, 2020.

31) Guterres. COVID-19 Threatens to Bring Back Unfair and Unequal Treatment of Working Women. Our World. May 6, 2020.

32) Krumholz, Harlan. Hydroxychloroquine and Azithromycin for COVID-19: Benefits TBD, Risks Clear. *Forbes*. April 10, 2020.

33) Rosenberg ES & Dufort EM. Association of Treatment with Hydroxychloroquine or Azithromycin with In-Hospital Mortality in Patients with COVID-19 in New York State. *JAMA*. May 11, 2020.

34) NIH (May 14, 2020). NIH begins clinical trial of hydroxychloroquine and azithromycin to treat COVID-19.

35) 7 News. "Vitamin D could be linked to COVID-10 survival, study suggests."

36) "Use of Ascorbic Acid in Patients with COVID-19." *Clinical trials.gov.*

37) "Recommendations for Investigational COVID-19 Convalescent Plasma." U.S. Food and Drug Administration. May 1, 2020.

38) Xu, X et al. Effective treatment of COVID-19 patients with Tocilizumab. Proceedings of the National Academy of Sciences of the United States of America. March 25, 2020.

39) Gillespie, C. "'Proning' is a common treatment for Coronavirus—Here's How it Works." April 21, 2020.

40) Hirsch, L. J.C. Penney plans to file for bankruptcy protection, sources say. *Msn Money.* May 15, 2020.

41) Langlois, S. "'The next big shoe to drop in the US economy' could hit in July." *Msn Money.* May 14, 2020.

42) Spivack, C. "New York's coronavirus eviction moratorium explained." May 11, 2020.

43) Caplinger, D. "There's a Surprise Tax Break in the Latest Relief Package Proposal." *MSN Money.* May 14, 2020.

44) Hawkins, D. et al. "Live updates: House passes $3 Trillion Relief Package; Texas Supreme Court Halts Voting by Mail Amid Coronavirus Pandemic." *The Washington Post.* May 16, 2020.

45) Hawkins, D. et al. "How Road Blocks Collide to Make Reopening Asian American Business Feel 'Just Impossible.'" *The Washington Post.* May 16, 2020.

46) "What You Need to Know About Coronavirus." *The Washington Post.* May 9, 2020.

47) "Your Weekend Briefing." *The New York Times.* May 17, 2020.

48) Watkins, A. "Top E.R. Doctor Who Treated Virus Patients Dies by Suicide." *The New York Times.* Aril 29, 2020.

49) "India coronavirus: Life-saving Covid-19 drugs sold on Delhi black market." *BBC.* Julu 7, 2020. Accessed from <https://news.yahoo.com/india-coronavirus-life-saving-covid-053953994.html>

50) "Coronaviurs: Taj Mahal reopens under new restrictions." Accessed from < https://en.as.com/en/2020/07/06/latest_news/1594068286_905788.html>

51) "South Africa to allocate last $2.6 billion of coronavirus stimulus." *AS.* July 7, 2020. Accessed on < https://en.as.com/en/2020/07/07/latest_news/1594147925_758306.html?omnil=resrelrecom>

52) Ferre-Sadurni L et al. "Does Cuomo Share Blame for the 6,200 Virus Deaths in N.Y. Nursing Homes?" *The New York Times.* July 8, 2020. Accessed from < https://www.nytimes.com/2020/07/08/nyregion/nursing-homes-deaths-coronavirus.html>

53) "What We do." *World Health Organization.* Accessed on May 19, 2020.

54) Klein B & Hansler J. "Trump halts WHO funding over handling of coronavirus outbreak." *CNN Politics.* April 15, 2020.

55) "Obesity: Facts, Figures, Guidelines." *DHHR.* Accessed on May 19, 2020.

56) Heart Disease Facts. *CDC.gov.* December 2, 2019.

57) "Can gargling or drinking hot liquids help prevent the coronavirus?" *WebMD.* May 19, 2020.

58) Ziady, H. "7 Things About COVID-19 That Worry Business Leaders the Most." *CNN Business.* May 19, 2020.

59) Silverman et al Navajo Nation surpasses New York state for the highest COVID-19 infection rate in the US. *CNN.* May 18, 2020.

60) Spells, A. Doctors Without Borders Dispatched to New Mexico to help the Navajo Nation. CNN *US.* May 11, 2020.

61) Tappe, A. "30 million Americans have filed initial unemployment claims since mid-March." *CNN Business.* April 30, 2020.

62) *DOL.gov News Release* (May 14, 2020). Unemployment Insurance Weekly Claims.

63) *U.S. Bureau of Labor Statistics (*May 19, 2020). Databases, Tables & Calculators by Subject.

64) Stanage, N. Five unanswered questions on COVID-19 and the 2020 election. *The Hill.* May 17, 2020. Accessed from < https://thehill.com/homenews/campaign/498134-five-unanswered-questions-on-covid-19-and-the-2020-election>

65) Valentic, S. 8 Quotes from the World Health Organization's COVID-19 Media Briefing. *EHS Today.* March 12, 2020. Accessed from <https://www.ehstoday.com/health/media-gallery/21126031/8-quotes-from-the-world-health-organizations-covid19-media-briefing>

66) May 18, 2020. Newswise Expert Panels on COVID-19 Pandemic: Notable excerpts, quotes, and videos available.

67) Magagnoli et al (April 21, 2020). Outcomes of hydroxychloroquine usage in United States veterans hospitalized with COVID-19. *MedRxiv.*

68) Hohman, M (May 19, 2020). Trump says he's taking hydroxychloroquine to prevent coronavirus- is it safe? *MSN Lifestyle.*

69) Locher, J. (April 21, 2020). More deaths, no benefit from malaria drug in VA virus study. *The Associated Press.*

70) *CDC.* If you are Pregnant, Breastfeeding, or Caring for Young Children. Accessed on May 19, 2020.

71) *CDC.* Cloth face coverings for children, parents, and other caregivers.

72) *The Economist.* (May 12, 2020). Can sports survive the COVID-19 pandemic without spectators?

73) May 20, 2020. China's New Outbreak Shows Signs the Virus Could be Changing. *Bloomberg.*

74) May 19, 2020. How China's Pledge to Give its Virus Vaccine Could Go. *Bloomberg.*

75) Hemenway-Forbes, M (April 14, 2020). Notable local Quotes on the COVID-19 pandemic.

76) The Emerging Link Between Obesity and COVID-19. *Health Matters.* Accessed on May 21, 2020.

77) (April 17, 2020). Clinical Characteristics of COVID-19 in New York City.

78) COVID-19: Why is it mild for some, deadly for others? An expert explores possible explanations for why some patients suffer serious complications. *Health Matters.*

79) Liu W et al (May 5, 2020). Analysis of Factors Associated with Disease Outcomes in Hospitalized Patients with 2019 Novel Coronavirus Disease. *China Med J (Engl).* 133(9): 1032-1038.

80) Eisenberg R (April 10, 2020). Is Working from Home the Future of Work?

81) McGinley L (April 28, 2020). Cancer Patients are nearly three times more likely to die of COVID-19, study says. *The Washington Post.*

82) Dai et al (April 28, 2020). Patients with cancer appear more vulnerable to SARS-CoV2- a multi-center study during the COVID-19 outbreak. *Cancer Discovery.*

83) Vaping and COVID-19: Can Vaping Increase Complications? *Health Matters*

84) Centers for Disease Control and Prevention. Coronavirus 2019: People Who Are at Higher Risk for Severe Illness.

85) Terry M (April 2, 2020). Compare: 1918 Spanish Influenza Pandemic Versus COVID-19.

86) Darlington S (May 24, 2020). Report: Brazil's indigenous people are dying at an alarming rate from COVID-19.

87) CDC Morbidity and Mortality Report (May 22, 2020). Decline in Child Vaccination Coverage During the COVID-19 Pandemic- Michigan Care Improvement Registry, May 2016-May 2020. 69(20); 630-631.

88) Thompson D (May 4, 2020). What is 'Contact Tracing' and How Does it Work?' *WebMD.*

89) *The Great Influenza.* John Barry. Penguin Books. New York, New York 2004.

90) Katz J and Sanger-Katz M (April 27, 2020). N.Y.C Deaths Reach 6 Times the Normal Level, Far More than Coronavirus Account Suggests. *The New York Times.* Accessed on May 28, 2020 from < https://www.nytimes.com/interactive/2020/04/27/upshot/coronavirus-deaths-new-york-city.html>

91) (May 27, 2020). An Incalculable Loss. *The New York Times*. Accessed on May 28, 2020 from << https://www.nytimes.com/interactive/2020/05/24/us/us-coronavirus-deaths-100000.html?campaign_id=154&emc=edit_cb_20200527&instance_id=18864&nl=coronavirus-briefing&regi_id=84718547&segment_id=29355&te=1&user_id=739bd6b20c937bef42adc6cbe5a068ce>>

92) Federal Reserve Bank of San Francisco. What is the difference between a recession and a depression? February 2007.

93) Fischer, S. Social media use spikes during pandemic. *Axios*. April 24, 2020.

94) Huston, C. Broadway businesses take a hit after theatre shutdown. *Broadway News*. March 25, 2020. Accessed from < https://broadwaynews.com/2020/03/25/broadway-businesses-take-a-hit-after-theater-shutdown/>

95) Headly, CW. New study reveals COVID-19 patients can remain immune for this amount of time. *Ladders*. May 28, 2020. Accessed from < https://www.theladders.com/career-advice/new-study-reveals-covid-19-patients-can-remain-immune-for-this-amount-of-time>

96) Popovich, N et al. "The World is Still Far from Herd Immunity for Coronavirus." *The New York Times*. May 28, 2020. Accessed from <https://www.nytimes.com/interactive/2020/05/28/upshot/coronavirus-herd-immunity.html.

97) Virus costs may linger for a decade. *Linked in*. 6/2/20. Accessed from < https://www.linkedin.com/feed/news/virus-costs-may-linger-for-a-decade-4134929>

98) Fleming, S. "New York is the epicenter of America's coronavirus outbreak. How is the city coping?" *World Economic Forum.* March 27, 2020.

99) Besheer, M. "As New York Looks to Heal from Coronavirus, Its Economy Falls Ill." April 16, 2020. Accessed from <voanews.com/covid-19-pandemic/new-york-looks-heal-coronavirus-its-economy-falls-ill>

100) "Responses to the COVID-19 Pandemic." *Prison Policy Initiative.* June 1, 2020. Accessed from <https://www.prisonpolicy.org/virus/viurses>

101) Roos, D. "Why the Second Wave of the Spanish Flu Was So Deadly." *History.* April 29, 2020. Accessed from < https://www.history.com/news/spanish-flu-second-wave-resurgence>

102) Zeitlen, M. "What Americans Need to Understand About the Swedish Coronavirus Experiment. *Gen.* May 11, 2020.

103) "The Employment Situation-April 2020." *Bureau of Labor Statistics.* May 8, 2020. Accessed from < https://www.bls.gov/news.release/pdf/empsit.pdf>

104) "Italy Coronavirus Cases." *Worldometer.* June 4, 2020. Accessed from < https://www.worldometers.info/coronavirus/country/italy/>

105) Belligoni, S. "5 Reasons the Coronavirus Hit Italy So Hard." *The Conversation.* March 26, 2020. Accessed from < https://theconversation.com/5-reasons-the-coronavirus-hit-italy-so-hard-134636>

106) Attia, P. "John Barry: 1918 Spanish flu pandemic- historical account, parallels to today, and lessons." *Peter Attia MD Podcast.* April 17, 2020.

107) Bay Area News Group. "George Floyd autopsy report, with cause of death and other factors. *The Mercury News.* June 5, 2020. Accessed from

<https://www.mercurynews.com/2020/06/05/read-george-floyd-autopsy-report-with-cause-of-death-and-other-factors/>

108) HealthDay. U.S. COVID-19 death rate is 1.3%, study finds. *Medical press.* May 8, 2020. Accessed from <https://medicalxpress.com/news/2020-05-covid-death.html>

109) Muchnick, J. "Rockland restaurants can reopen June 9; here's where to go for outdoor dining." *MSN Lifestyle.* June 8, 2020. Accessed from <https://www.msn.com/en-us/travel/news/rockland-restaurants-can-reopen-june-9-heres-where-to-go-for-outdoor-dining/ar=BB15cDac>

110) New York State. "What You Need to Know." *Information on Novel Coronavirus.* June 8, 2020. Accessed from <https://coronavirus.health.ny.gov/home?ocid=eventhub

111) Hoff T. "COVID-19 fallout: How will other needed care be provided during the pandemic?" *Medical Economics.* March 24, 2020. Accessed from <medicaleconomics.com/news/covid-19-fallout-how-will-other-needed-care-be-provided-during-pandemic>

112) Adams B. "Lilly starts second COVID-19 antibody test with partner Junshi Biosciences, eyes combo trials." *Biotech.* June 8, 2020. Accessed from <fiercebiotech.com/biotech/lilly-starts-second-covid-19-antibody-test-partner-junshi-biosciences-eyes-combo-trials>

113) "Complications Coronavirus Can Cause." *WebMD.* Accessed from <https://www.webmd.com/lung/coronavirus

114) New York State Information on Novel Coronavirus Webinar. "Weekly Health Provider Webinar." June 10, 2020. Accessed from < https://coronavirus.health.ny.gov/weekly-health-provider-webinar>

115) "2009 H1N1 Pandemic." *Centers for Disease Control and Prevention.* June 11, 2019. Accessed from <cdc.gov/flu/pandemic-resources/2009-h1n1=pandemic.html.>

116) Huang P. "Nothing Like SARS: Researchers Warn the Coronavirus Will Not Fade Away Anytime Soon." NPR. June 11, 2020. Accessed from <Npr.org.>

117) McKenna S. "What COVID-19 Antibody Tests Can and Cannot Tell Us." Scientific American. May 5, 2020. Accessed from < https://www.scientificamerican.com/article/what-covid-19-antibody-tests-can-and-cannot-tell-us/>

118) Zagaria ME. "Sarcopenia: Loss of Muscle Mass in Older Adults." U.S. Pharmacist. September 20, 2010. Accessed from < https://www.uspharmacist.com/article/sarcopenia-loss-of-muscle-mass-in-older-adults>

119) Groth L. "This Coming Epidemic Could be Deadlier Than COVID-19, Warn Experts." *MSN Lifestyle.* June 15, 2020. Accessed from <https://www.msn.com/en-us/health/medical/this-coming-epidemic-could-be-deadlier-than-covid-19-warns-experts/ar-BB15vqqo?ocid=spartandhp.>

120) Raphael T. "How COVID-19 Has Set Back the Fight Against Cancer." *MSN Lifestyle.* June 15, 2020. Accessed from <https://www.msn.com/en-us/medical/how-covid-19-has-set-back-the-fight-against-cancer/ar-BB15uXS?ocid=spartandhp.

121) Reinicke C. "'Painfully evident' damage: Deutsche Bank now thinks the US economy will shrink by nearly 40% in the 2nd quarter following coronavirus lockdowns." *Business Insider.* May 11, 2020. Accessed from < https://www.businessinsider.com/us-economy-gdp-will-shrink-second-quarter-deutsche-bank-coronavirus-2020-5>

122) Stuplin C. "Seasonality will "eventually" play a role in COVID-19 transmission." *Helio.* May 2, 2020. Accessed from < https://www.healio.com/news/infectious-disease/20200501/seasonality-will-eventually-play-a-role-in-covid19-transmission>

123) Rabin RC. "Nearly All Patients Hospitalized with COVID-19 Had Chronic Health Issues, Study Finds." *The New York Times.* April 23, 2020. Accessed from < https://www.nytimes.com/2020/04/23/health/coronavirus-patients-risk.html>

124) Mueller B et al. "Common Drug Reduces Coronavirus Deaths, Scientists Report." *The New York Times.* June 16, 2020. Accessed from <https://www.nytimes.com/2020/06/16/world/europe/dexamethasone-coronavirus-covid.html?action=click&pgtype=Article&state=default&module=STYLN_daily_question_block&region=body&context=storylines_faq>

125) Henley J. "Just 7.3% of Stockholm had COVID-19 antibodies by end of April, study shows." *The Guardian.* May 21, 2020. Accessed from https://www/google.com/amp/s/amp.theguardian

126) "Eli Lilly COVID-19 treatment could be authorized for use as soon as September, chief scientist says." June 10, 2020. Accessed from <https://www.cnbc.com/20>

127) Gal S. "American Resilience: How 5 industries bounced back from 9/11, hurricanes, and the Great Recession- and what their success can teach us about hope after the coronavirus." *Business Insider*. July 3, 2020. Accessed from < https://www.businessinsider.com/american-resilience-how-restaurants-airlines-real-estate-recovered-from-disasters-2020-7>

128) Woodward A. "The US has run out of time and excuses. Now we'll be forced to watch thousands die of coronavirus." *Business Insider*. July 10, 2020. Accessed from <https://www.businessinsider.com/coronavirus-rising-cases-hospitalizations-herald-surge-in-us-deaths-2020-7?utm_source=notification&utm_medium=referral>

129) Cave D. "New Zealand Lifts Lockdown as It Declares Virus Eliminated, For Now." *The New York Times*. June 8, 2020. Accessed from < https://www.nytimes.com/2020/06/08/world/australia/new-zealand-coronavirus-ardern.html>

130) AJMC Staff. "A Timeline of Coronavirus Developments in 2020." *AJMC*. July 3, 2020. Accessed on < https://www.ajmc.com/focus-of-the-week/a-timeline-of-covid19-developments-in-2020///?p=4>

131) Tremaine J. "Disney World reopens: Take an inside look at the Magic Kingdom today." *CNN Travel*. July 12, 2020. Accessed from < https://www.cnn.com/travel/article/disney-world-magic-kingdom-reopens/index.html>

132) Barnes B. "Disney World Opens its Gates, With Virus Numbers Rising." *The New York Times*. July 11, 2020. Accessed from < https://www.nytimes.com/2020/07/11/business/florida-coronavirus-disney-world-reopening.html?campaign_id=9&emc=edit_nn_20200712&instance_id=20247&nl=th

e-morning&regi_id=111579486&segment_id=33206&te=1&user_id=1a5d64ae2d5b28add21bf828ab0c47fe>

133) "Guidelines: Opening Up America Again." *WhiteHouse.gov*. Accessed from < https://www.whitehouse.gov/openingamerica/>

134) "Trump gives in to the mask but takes new risks with schools." *CNN politics*. July 12, 2020. Accessed from < https://www.cnn.com/2020/07/12/politics/trump-mask-coronavirus-schools-reopening/index.html>

135) Jewett C et al. "Exclusive: Nearly 600—And Counting—US Health Workers Have Died of COVID-19." *Kaiser Health News*. June 6, 2020. Accessed from < https://khn.org/news/exclusive-investigation-nearly-600-and-counting-us-health-workers-have-died-of-covid-19/>

136) "COVID-19 Data." *NYC Health*. Accessed from < Katz J and Sanger-Katz M (April 27, 2020). N.Y.C Deaths Reach 6 Times the Normal Level, Far More than Coronavirus Account Suggests. *The New York Times*. Accessed on May 28, 2020 from < https://www.nytimes.com/interactive/2020/04/27/upshot/coronavirus-deaths-new-york-city.html>

www.ingramcontent.com/pod-product-compliance
Lightning Source LLC
Chambersburg PA
CBHW080451220526

45465CB00006B/2229